MOTIVATIONAL INTERVIEWING
WITH OFFENDERS

Applications of Motivational Interviewing

Stephen Rollnick, William R. Miller,
and Theresa B. Moyers, Series Editors

www.guilford.com/AMI

Since the publication of Miller and Rollnick's classic *Motivational Interviewing*, now in its third edition, MI has been widely adopted as a tool for facilitating change. This highly practical series includes general MI resources as well as books on specific clinical contexts, problems, and populations. Each volume presents powerful MI strategies that are grounded in research and illustrated with concrete, "how-to-do-it" examples.

Motivational Interviewing in Health Care:
Helping Patients Change Behavior
Stephen Rollnick, William R. Miller, and Christopher C. Butler

Motivational Interviewing with Adolescents and Young Adults
Sylvie Naar and Mariann Suarez

Motivational Interviewing in Social Work Practice
Melinda Hohman

Motivational Interviewing in the Treatment of Anxiety
Henny A. Westra

Motivational Interviewing, Third Edition: Helping People Change
William R. Miller and Stephen Rollnick

Motivational Interviewing in Groups
Christopher C. Wagner and Karen S. Ingersoll, with Contributors

Motivational Interviewing in the Treatment
of Psychological Problems, Second Edition
Hal Arkowitz, William R. Miller, and Stephen Rollnick, Editors

Motivational Interviewing in Diabetes Care
Marc P. Steinberg and William R. Miller

Motivational Interviewing in Nutrition and Fitness
Dawn Clifford and Laura Curtis

Motivational Interviewing in Schools:
Conversations to Improve Behavior and Learning
Stephen Rollnick, Sebastian G. Kaplan, and Richard Rutschman

Motivational Interviewing with Offenders:
Engagement, Rehabilitation, and Reentry
Jill D. Stinson and Michael D. Clark

Motivational Interviewing and CBT:
Combining Strategies for Maximum Effectiveness
Sylvie Naar and Steven A. Safren

Building Motivational Interviewing Skills, Second Edition:
A Practitioner Workbook
David B. Rosengren

MOTIVATIONAL INTERVIEWING WITH OFFENDERS

Engagement, Rehabilitation, and Reentry

JILL D. STINSON
MICHAEL D. CLARK

Series Editors' Note by
Stephen Rollnick, William R. Miller,
and Theresa B. Moyers

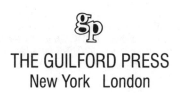

THE GUILFORD PRESS
New York   London

Library of Congress Cataloging-in-Publication Data

Names: Stinson, Jill D., author. | Clark, Michael D. (Michael Duane), 1955–
  author.
Title: Motivational interviewing with offenders : engagement, rehabilitation,
  and reentry / Jill D. Stinson, Michael D. Clark.
Description: New York, NY : Guilford Press, [2017] | Series: Applications of
  motivational interviewing | Includes bibliographical references and index.
Identifiers: LCCN 2017000494| ISBN 9781462529872 (pbk. : alk. paper) | ISBN
  9781462529889 (hardcover : alk. paper)
Subjects: LCSH: Social work with sex offenders. | Motivational interviewing.
  | Sex offenders—Rehabilitation. | Sex offenders—Counseling of.
Classification: LCC HV6556 .S75 2017 | DDC 365/.661—dc23
LC record available at *https://lccn.loc.gov/2017000494*

To my family, without whom this would not be possible
—J. D. S.

With thanks and gratitude to
Frances, Rebecca, Brian, Steven, and Molly
—M. D. C.

ABOUT THE AUTHORS

Jill D. Stinson, PhD, is Assistant Professor and Director of Clinical Training in the Department of Psychology at East Tennessee State University. She previously served as an administrator and sex offender treatment coordinator at Fulton State Hospital, a maximum- and intermediate-security forensic mental health hospital in Missouri. Her research and publications focus on sex offenders with serious mental illness, the role of self-regulation in treatment of personality and severe behavior disorders, and the impact of early childhood trauma in high-risk psychiatric and offender populations. Dr. Stinson is an active member of the Association for the Treatment of Sexual Abusers and an associate editor of *Sexual Abuse: A Journal of Research and Treatment.*

Michael D. Clark, MSW, is Director of the Center for Strength-Based Strategies, a Michigan-based training and technical assistance group. His interests lie in the application of strength-based and motivational practices for marginalized, court-mandated populations. Mr. Clark served for 16 years as a probation officer and a court magistrate in Lansing, Michigan. He is a board member of the International Association for Correctional and Forensic Psychology and served on an expert panel for the United Nations Office on Drugs and Crime in Vienna, Austria. A member of the Motivational Interviewing Network of Trainers, he delivers MI training in blended learning formats to probation officers, reentry staff, juvenile justice professionals, and addiction counselors across the United States. His website is *www.buildmotivation.com.*

SERIES EDITORS' NOTE

Motivational interviewing (MI) seems to find a natural home in serving society's most marginalized people, and surely offenders have been among them. Attitudes toward offenders are changing, with a gradual shift away from ineffective retribution toward restoration, rehabilitation, and active engagement in the process of change. External controls are substantial during incarceration, but people's own motivations play a greater role in governing their behavior and life course once they have returned to the community, as most offenders do. Engaging such control from within can buffer the predictable rebound that can occur upon release from external controls.

In this groundbreaking volume Jill Stinson and Michael Clark describe how the collaborative, empathic, and affirming style of MI lends itself to a restorative approach. MI presents a fresh new approach to facilitating offender engagement and meaningful change. Drawing on their long experience and expertise with offender rehabilitation and reentry, the authors explain the applicability of MI all the way from shifting perceptions of offenders to promoting culture change in offender systems. They deftly balance a positive approach to change with responsibility for public safety. In the end, these two concerns are usually the same, because effective change in offending behavior is a vital element in protecting public welfare.

Over recent years, criminal justice, correctional, and forensic mental health professionals and systems have slowly shifted from an adversarial to a more engaging and collaborative approach. Some have already done so and others are en route, conscious that ultimately it is offenders themselves who make choices about their own role and behavior in institutions as well as in the community. To be sure, some limits can be set and consequences enforced, but ultimately people still make their own decisions. That autonomous choice cannot be taken away from a person. MI is a way of exploring that decision-making process and evoking the person's own motivations for prosocial change.

So be prepared for some stimulating and thought-provoking reading. MI is a learnable style of conversation that can be used in institutions, in formal supervision in the community, and even in passing hallway conversations. You may recognize some of what you read here as familiar, something that you already know at some level to be true. Other aspects of MI may seem surprising, even jolting. Settle in as these two seasoned professionals tell the story of this approach and how it can change offenders, providers, and systems. We hope that much of what you find here will prove both useful and rewarding in your own work.

STEPHEN ROLLNICK
WILLIAM R. MILLER
THERESA B. MOYERS

ACKNOWLEDGMENTS

So many people were instrumental in the development and completion of this text. Our profound thanks to Bill Miller, Steve Rollnick, and Theresa Moyers for their vast knowledge and skill in teaching MI to the eager learner. Thanks also to those who so thoughtfully provided their feedback, support, and examples as we sought to incorporate real-world experiences from MI professionals: Julio Acevedo, April Aguilar, Rob Axsen, Rob Bibbianni, Steve Brazill, Liz Cavillo, Carl Ake Farbring, Rhonda Gilbert, Ray Gingerich, Betty Hanna, Don Keeler, Adrienne Lindsey, Marc Marquez, Ken McMaster, David Prescott, Todd Roberts, Ron Skidmore, and Dee Dee Stout. Thank you to Lydia Eisenbrandt, Kelcey Hall, and Carrie LeMay for compiling materials for this text. And lest we forget, it does take a village—thanks go to Ruthie Brooks, Sarah Dixon, Lee Ann McVay, Michele Moser, Megan Quinn, Victoria Wells, and so many others who have given their gifts of time and encouragement in seeing this project through. We also want to especially acknowledge Scott T. Walters, Ray Gingerich, and Melissa L. Meltzer, who co-authored with Michael D. Clark the DOJ/NIC monograph (Walters, Clark, Gingerich, & Meltzer, 2007) that formed the basis for Chapter 12. Your camaraderie and your contributions are contained herein with deep appreciation. Finally, we would like to thank those in the field of corrections and criminal justice who kept the mission of rehabilitation alive during the dark decades of punishment. Your humane and compassionate spirit and your dedication to respectful, client-centered approaches have paved the way for our field to find its way back into the light.

CONTENTS

1. A New Approach   1

2. The Spirit of Motivational Interviewing   15

3. The Art of Listening   31

4. The Art of Interviewing   44

5. Engaging: The Relational Foundation   62

6. Engaging: The Relationship in Practice   75

7. Focusing and Preparing for Change   95

8. Focusing in Practice   108

9. Evoking: Moving toward Change   125

10. Evoking in Practice　　　　　　　　　140

11. Developing a Plan　　　　　　　　　164

12. Resistance Reexamined　　　　　　　180

13. The Rise of Motivational Interviewing　　199

14. Implementation and Sustainability　　211

15. Considerations, Cautions, and Comments　231

References　　　　　　　　　　　　243

Index　　　　　　　　　　　　　256

MOTIVATIONAL INTERVIEWING WITH OFFENDERS

CHAPTER 1

A NEW APPROACH

Imagine for a moment the following headlines in your local or national news:

> "Hundreds of ex-cons get jobs, lead normal, uneventful lives"
> "Community welcomes back former inmates"
> "Prisons sit empty as community treatment programs thrive"
> "Majority of violent offenders don't reoffend, not a threat to society"

This is vastly different from the reality, is it not? Instead, a frightened public decries the failure of our systems to prevent crime and appropriately sanction offenders. Prisons and harsh offender policies become the norm, and communities seek ways to prohibit former offenders from returning. As these unlikely headlines demonstrate, there are marked discrepancies among the science of offender rehabilitation, the practice of those who work with offenders, and the expectations and beliefs of a concerned public. These differences are most obvious to those who work with offenders each day within the criminal justice system, residential and community corrections, forensic mental health systems, and risk management agencies like probation and parole. Within these agencies, we struggle with the shared goals of promoting community safety, improving offender rehabilitation, and facilitating successful reentry outcomes. These goals require a careful balance between responsibilities—the responsibility of the offender for his or her own actions and behavior, and the responsibility of those charged with reentry planning and risk management. It can be a precarious balancing act.

How do you do this? How can you balance these responsibilities in such a way as to promote public safety while still fulfilling your obligations to the offender to provide effective services? Historically, two goals have been at the forefront in offender rehabilitation and risk management. *Compliance* is a pragmatic goal, dependent on the assumption that offenders who comply with supervisory and legal rules will be successful in refraining from continued criminal behavior. Attention and effort are focused mostly on securing and maintaining an offender's compliance with treatment, with surveillance and reporting requirements, and with prosocial lifestyle supports. Put simply, you want offenders to follow the rules, and when they do, you feel assured that they will be successful and safe. It is a short-term acquiescence to power and authority that may not extend beyond a single meeting or a term of supervision. Compliance communicates a brief stabilization of behavior, but one that may not generalize to other, more long-term contexts.

A second and perhaps more important goal, however, is *behavior change*. This involves a combination of motivation, self-evaluation, and the development of new behaviors. Underlying the goal of behavior change are assumptions that an offender must be motivated and capable of change, and that such change will be in a positive, prosocial direction. Lasting behavior change is motivated by self-important values. Such change is self-directed, and in offender systems, the goal of change is viewed with some skepticism and trepidation. It is a complicated, lengthy, and often less immediately visible process. Further, an offender's ability to change relies on not just the offender but also other people, support systems, and social factors interactively working together. At any point, conditions may facilitate behavior change or hinder it.

One may mistakenly think of these two goals as independent, though they are not. Compliance is more observable and easily measured. It can also be more easily systematized and applied with less individual variability—all of these are things that make compliance much more attainable from the perspective of large, bureaucratic systems. However, the reality is that one cannot achieve compliance without behavior change, or at least, not in the long term. If one expects compliance without change, then an offender will comply only so long as he or she is being closely monitored and directly supported. Once supervision and support systems are removed, the individual's behavior will return to its former state, which may mean a lifestyle involving criminal behavior. Thus, we must critically evaluate our focus in working with offenders.

MOTIVATIONAL INTERVIEWING

Though specific roles may vary, the primary aim of those who work with offenders is to promote meaningful change in those who have committed criminal offenses. Enter motivational interviewing, or "MI." This approach (Miller & Rollnick, 1991, 2002, 2013) is a way of communicating with people about change. It first emerged from work with addictions but has since widened its reach, becoming a favored approach for use with populations in a variety of settings (Burke, Arkowitz, & Dunn, 2002), including criminal justice agencies (Birgden, 2004; McMurran, 2002; Farrall, 2002), probation (Walters, Clark, Gingerich, & Meltzer, 2007; Clark, 2005; Ginsburg, Mann, Rotgers, & Weekes, 2002; Harper & Hardy, 2000; Miller, 1999), and corrections (Anstiss, Polaschek, & Wilson, 2011). Broadly, this growth in the use of MI parallels a move toward the "business of behavior change" in corrections and criminal justice (Clark, Walters, Gingerich, & Meltzer, 2006). But specifically, it means agencies across North America and the world have begun to incorporate MI within their offender treatment and reentry services, for both mental health or specialty service professionals as well as direct line staff. More than 30 nations have adopted MI for use within their courts, prisons, and community corrections and supervision agencies, as is evidenced by the availability of trainers and trainings in multiple languages and locations (*www.motivationalinterviewing.org*). And at the 2010 United Nations Congress on Crime Prevention and Criminal Justice in Salvador, Brazil—a meeting that has been held every 5 years since World War II—the implementation of MI in correctional systems emerged as a key topic.

Why such growing interest in MI? Perhaps most evident is this: *It works.* As would be expected from its early roots in substance abuse treatment, MI has received its greatest empirical support from research on engaging substance users in treatment and improving their treatment outcomes (e.g., Apodaca & Longabaugh, 2009; Jensen et al., 2001; Vasilaki, Hosier, & Cox, 2006). Similarly, MI has been effectively used to supplement or enhance treatment engagement and progress in offender populations in prisons and community probation agencies (e.g., Farbring & Johnson, 2008; Harper & Hardy, 2000; McMurran, 2009; Walters et al., 2007; Walters, Vader, Nguyen, Harris, & Eells, 2010), as well as juvenile justice populations (Feldstein & Ginsburg, 2007; Sinha, Easton, Renee-Aubin, & Carroll, 2003; Slavet et al., 2005), domestic violence offenders (e.g., Dia, Simmons, Oliver, & Cooper, 2009; Kistenmacher

& Weiss, 2008; Murphy & Maiuro, 2009; Musser & Murphy, 2009; Musser, Semiatin, Taft, & Murphy, 2008; Rasmussen, Hughes, & Murray, 2008), and offenders with coexisting substance abuse and mental health problems (Mendel & Hipkins, 2002). In addition to these applications, numerous studies have demonstrated the impact of MI on treatment compliance and adherence (e.g., Lundahl & Burke, 2009) and increasing engagement in treatment for persons with serious mental illness (e.g., Arkowitz, Miller, & Rollnick, 2015), both of which are relevant to offender work.

These studies of offender populations tell us that MI works, though our goal here is not to exhaustively review the evidence of its effectiveness. Rather, we want to discuss other reasons for increased use of MI among offender service agencies. We have identified five additional factors to consider as you read this text, setting the stage for a shift in your thinking and practice with offender clients.

1. *MI aligns your department or agency with evidence-based practice.* MI was introduced in the early 1980s and has since been identified as an evidence-based practice (Substance Abuse and Mental Health Services Administration, 2008). Empirical study of MI suggests that certain types of brief counseling interactions are as beneficial as more lengthy interventions, and that a certain kind of provider style more effectively elicits change. A person who talks about the benefits of change is more likely to make that change, whereas a person who argues and defends the status quo is more likely to continue his or her problematic behavior (Miller & Rollnick, 2013). MI helps people connect the need for change to something they care about, which helps internalize the change process. It moves away from confrontation and toward collaboration, wherein a provider and client are each responsible for parts of the change process. That these elements are empirically supported and align with best practices for multiple client problem areas makes them particularly relevant for those who work with offenders.

Funding allocated for institutional and community-based offender service agencies is often subject to political and economic trends. Clear and Frost (2013) describe U.S. correctional budgets that in recent decades doubled or tripled (or more) following politically fueled mandated sentencing laws and other increases in sanctioning. This excess came to an abrupt end with the onset of economic recession in 2008. Sharp decreases in funding across countries in North America and other parts of the world have been felt across offender service systems, including not only corrections but probation and parole, forensic mental health, and diversionary programs. As a result, offender programs have far fewer resources with which to demonstrate effective rehabilitation and reentry practices. Those that fail to produce positive results risk losing even more of their scant funding. Failure can no longer be excused by "but we've always done it that way." Perhaps now more than ever, offender programs need to be developed based on evidence rather than ideology. Our work must have a clear grounding in science to continue to receive funding and support.

While having an adequate budget is ideal, money alone does not drive your efforts—effectiveness is paramount. Until only the past two decades, criminal justice suffered from a lack of proven methods for reducing offender recidivism (Bonta & Andrews, 2003). Today, it is almost unimaginable that the field ever operated without practice methods that were studied and empirically validated through rigorous science. Science-based methods for offender work have been propelled by multiple streams of interest, united by the "Evidence-Based Policy and Practice" initiative from the National Institute of Corrections (Bogue et al., 2004; Guevera & Solomon, 2009). This initiative named eight principles of effective intervention to reduce the risk of recidivism, among which MI was prominently cited in principle 2: "*Enhance Intrinsic Motivation*—Research strongly suggests that 'motivational interviewing' techniques, rather than persuasion tactics, effectively enhance motivation for initiating and maintaining behavior change" (Guevera & Solomon, 2009, p. 13).

Within this text, our goal is to lend substance to that recommendation by describing the benefits of integrating motivational strategies into offender work, and by providing best-practice examples of effective MI from the field.

But how does this fit with other empirically supported practices for offender rehabilitation and reentry? Any review of evidence-based practice in corrections and criminal justice invariably includes the risk–needs–responsivity (RNR) model (Andrews, Bonta, & Hoge, 1990; Bonta & Andrews, 2007). This model recommends that the level of service should match an offender's risk of reoffending, that offender agencies should assess an offender's criminogenic needs (i.e., dynamic risk factors) and focus treatment efforts on those issues, and that treatment should be matched to an offender's learning style, strengths and abilities, and inherent motivation to assist positive behavior change. This model clarifies who we should treat (i.e., risk), what we should do in treatment (i.e., needs), and most importantly, *how we should treat* (i.e., responsivity).

The RNR model brought renewed optimism to the field. After decades adrift, this method demonstrated reduced recidivism in an accessible and practical way, providing much-needed empirically grounded and scientifically confirmed outcomes. However, the RNR model is not a perfect solution (e.g., Polaschek, 2012). The most oft-cited critiques are that it can be more about programs than people, and that there's a lack of clear guidance for day-to-day implementation of the RNR principles across diverse programs and offender groups (Polaschek, 2012). And it is true that one must retain a focus on the person in order to apply any empirically based model effectively. Even the best approaches will fail if the offender is disinterested and does not want to participate. Start with client engagement, or forget starting at all. Bonta, Rugge, Scott, Bourgon, and Yessine (2008) have echoed problems with integrity of service delivery, particularly with regard to applying the principles of risk, need, and responsivity. However, MI can then provide not only an opportunity for empirically based service delivery, but also a method for increasing individualized treatment planning and enhancing service implementation in accordance with the fundamental principles of RNR.

Realizing that offender engagement is a critical first step, administrators and researchers alike have found that MI can transform mechanical and depersonalized offender models and add important core counseling skills. As a result, the most widely accepted RNR programs within the last decade have also taught MI as an important component (e.g., EPICS, University of Cincinnati Correctional Institute; STARR, Robinson, VanBenschoten, Alexander, & Lowenkamp, 2011; see Gleicher et al., 2013) to better facilitate a climate of behavior change.

> *A person who talks about the benefits of change is more likely to make that change.*

2. MI gets you back in the game of behavior change. To be about compliance—the traditional goal of offender rehabilitation and reentry—is not enough. Our work must be about fostering lasting changes in offender behavior. Trends in offender management, however, have misdirected us from this goal. While it is true that you can never "make" anyone change, or even want to change, what you can do is help people find their intrinsic motivation to improve themselves, have better lives, and make decisions that they value. This shift in thinking puts you in a position to be more than watchdogs or gatekeepers. You are then positioned to understand offenders and work with them to identify goals and barriers to change. Here, motivation is vital. You must understand a person's motivation before you can help him or her move forward.

Historically, motivation has been viewed as a more-or-less fixed characteristic of offenders. That is, an offender presents with a certain motivational "profile," and until that individual is ready for change, there is little that you can do to influence his or her choices and behaviors. Under this model, you work with the offender to enforce the orders of the court but are not necessarily an active participant in the offender's behavior change process. For example, a probation officer might describe his or her role this way:

> "The defendant and his lawyer negotiate for the judge to consider probation supervision (and conditions) in lieu of jail time. In our initial meeting and throughout our work together, I tell the probationer what is expected of him and make it clear what the penalties will be should he fail to comply. We have regular meetings to verify that he is making progress on his conditions, and I answer any questions he might have. If he breaks the law or shows poor progress, I see to it that appropriate sanctions are applied. Throughout the process, the probationer is well aware of the behavior that might send him to jail, and if he ends up there, it's his own behavior that gets him there."

This summary reflects the thoughts of an officer who is essentially removed from the change process, relegated to the role of an observer. Others who work with this population may feel the same sense of distance from the offender's efforts to change. However, there is a fair amount one can do to influence an offender's chances of success. But what you need is a mechanism through which to involve yourself in the process. MI thus puts you back in the game of behavior change.

In doing so, MI fundamentally changes what we talk about. No longer are we passive observers of our clients' decisions, focusing our discussions on rules and requirements and hoping that they will comply. Instead, we are active facilitators of growth and change, and as such, we emphasize this in our conversations with offenders. Ample evidence suggests that people can talk themselves into change, as well as talk themselves out of it (e.g., Walters, Ogle, & Martin, 2002). You play a crucial role in this process. For instance, linguistics research shows that the speech of the provider sets the tone for the speech of the client, which in turn influences the ultimate outcome (e.g., Amrhein, Miller, Yahne, Palmer, & Fulcher, 2003). Particular statements and questions, in addition to a certain provider style, predict decisions to change even during brief conversations. Offenders may come in with a certain range of readiness, but what we say beyond that makes a difference in how the person speaks, thinks, and ultimately chooses to act.

MI is about noticing and eliciting change talk, or self-motivational speech. Empirical research examining the effectiveness of MI has spotlighted this effect. Linguists have studied the speech content of brief motivational sessions (i.e., the actual words spoken between provider and client) looking for determinants of positive behavior change (Amrhein et al., 2003). Five categories of motivational speech were identified: desire, ability, reason, need, and commitment language. Later work included activation and taking steps, denoting different phases of change talk and change efforts. These categories have been summarized by Miller and Rollnick (2013) and are discussed further in Chapter 9. While we may understand that these concepts relate to change, we may be unused to listening carefully for them in our everyday interactions with offenders. Not every dimension must be voiced for important behavior change to start, though change talk is generally what most predicts behavior change.

In addition to this, MI changes *who* does the talking. MI teaches you to strategically steer a conversation in a particular direction, such as toward change talk or commitment to change, but such steering is of little value if you are unable to move the conversation forward. One may feel pressure to do this and consequently end up working harder than the offender. Consider, for example, the findings of a recent study of probation officers (Clark, 2005): When office appointments between offenders and their assigned probation officers were audio- and videotaped, in the average 15-minute visit, the officers spent far more time talking than did the offenders. In one instance, the officer spoke more than 70% of the time. In a similar interview, another officer spoke more than twice as much as the offender. Quantity does not beget quality, and these officers may be talking themselves out of effectiveness. The more you talk, the less opportunity there is for the offender to talk and think about change. Instead, you can use strategies to get the offender talking and engaged in the change process. Thus, MI has much to offer offender agencies in the way of moving clients toward change.

> *Our work must be about fostering lasting changes in offender behavior.*

3. MI prepares offenders for the work of change. People need to prepare for change. This is as true for offenders as it is for the rest of us.

We are seldom taught to prepare people for change. Instead, we jump to problem solving, planning, encouraging productive talk, and the like, ignoring or bypassing the need to orient to change work. Getting the offender to talk is a first step, followed by preparation for change. MI trains us in basic listening and engagement strategies to help with this process, many of which we will discuss in Chapters 3, 4, 5, and 6. Such methods help the offender approach change in a more planful and informed way, allowing you to gather better information in order to facilitate the overall process.

In Figure 1.1 we illustrate some of the markers that help to determine whether the client is moving toward change.

Clients may have a range of actions moving them either toward or away from change. As you think about how to prepare them for active commitment and behavior change, you must not only assess where they are on this continuum, but also establish for them that such a continuum exists. The client must recognize his or her own position toward a desired or needed life change.

Prior literature has examined the stages of change, first introduced by Prochaska and DiClemente (1982, 1992) with regard to observed change processes in persons involved in smoking cessation efforts. In brief, these authors identified five nonlinear stages through which people move as they are contemplating a behavioral or life change. First is

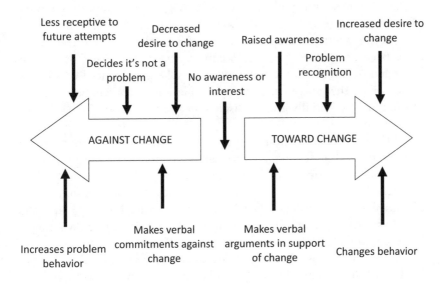

FIGURE 1.1. Orienting clients to the continuum of change.

precontemplation, a stage in which people find it difficult to recognize or accept a need to change. Individuals may be unaware of the problem and feel comfortable with the status quo. Despite negative consequences or efforts from others to precipitate change, they lack insight into their own contribution to the problem and may blame others or deny the need to change. The second is *contemplation,* or the point at which the person becomes ambivalent, or of mixed feelings about the problem (to be discussed further in Chapter 7). It is now that the person begins feeling uncomfortable about the status quo but has not yet reached the point of making a decision about what to do. *Preparation* is the stage during which the person is inclined toward change but may not yet have made a firm decision. This stage may include identifying goals, defining small next steps, or seeking additional information about the desired change. *Action* is the stage on which we focus the greatest amount of our attention, in which the person has taken initial steps toward change and evidences noticeable changes in attitude and behavior. Finally, we have *maintenance,* where the individual has been successful in making necessary changes and is now ready to work toward sustaining them and avoiding or planning for potential setbacks.

The stages of change are a useful way of conceptualizing the ways in which one could or should interact with persons who are faced with future changes. They illustrate how persons may need to orient themselves at various points along the way, or what may be required of them as they consider and implement change. MI, while distinctly separate from these stages of change (Miller & Rollnick, 2009), would have you become acutely attuned and responsive to clients' fluid needs over time. Because offenders are often considering changes that have been suggested or imposed externally, there may be greater need to address persons in earlier stages (i.e., precontemplation or contemplation), and this requires potentially greater discussion and orientation to the change process itself.

MI uses a combination of skills and strategies to not only initiate conversations about change, but to help orient and guide the client as he or she makes important decisions about change. This is accomplished through the use of questions, reflections, and check-in summaries (all discussed in greater detail in Chapter 6) to assist both you and the offender with understanding the nature of the problem and how it might be best approached. For some examples, see Box 1.1.

These questions, meant to provoke interest in change, will also likely encourage more productive talk about change. Offenders have mixed feelings, and since what may happen to them is not always certain,

---

BOX 1.1. ASK QUESTIONS THAT RAISE THE CLIENT'S INTEREST IN TALKING ABOUT CHANGE

Drawbacks of Current Behavior

- "What concerns do you have about your drug use?"
- "What concerns does your wife have about your drug use?"
- "What has your drug use cost you?"

Benefits of Change

- "If you went ahead and took care of that class, how would that make things better for you?"
- "You talk a lot about your family. How would finding a job benefit your family?"
- "How would that make things better for your kids?"

Desire to Change

- "How badly do you want that?"
- "How does that make you feel?"
- "How would that make you feel differently?"

Perceived Ability to Change

- "How would you do that if you wanted to?"
- "What would that take?"
- "If you did decide to change, what makes you think you could do it?"

Commitments the Offender Will Make

- "How are you going to do that?"
- "What will that look like?"
- "How are you going to make sure that happens?"

---

they need every opportunity to talk and think about positive behavior change. Ideally, this process reinforces movement toward change: Your questions evoke change talk, the offender responds with positive statements, you reflect and reinforce such statements, and the client continues to elaborate and solidify his or her commitment. Thus MI has become a standard of practice with offenders in order to help them move toward the commitments they may make. And in doing this, you save yourself time. By targeting your talk toward more productive and meaningful exploration, you help people move more quickly toward their values and also reduce frustration. Research on MI in health care settings (Knight, McGowen, Dickens, & Bundy, 2006) has shown this approach not only to elicit change but to *save providers time.*

**4. MI *shifts the balance of responsibility, making us agents of change rather than responsible for change.* Typically, those who work with offenders assume a great deal of responsibility for the offender's behavior, along with responsibility for whether or not it ultimately changes. Such assumptions promote the illusion of control over the outcome. But they also imply that both failures and successes are attributable to your own skill, decision making, or influence. This carries significant implications for how one views the change process for offenders, perhaps placing more attention on agency staff members than may be warranted.

The skills and the services provided to the offender represent only part of the picture, and not necessarily the most important part. Research finds that long-term change is more likely to occur for *intrinsic* reasons (Deci & Ryan, 1985). Quite often, what one assumes would motivate the offender simply does not. MI would have you discover the things that are valued by the individual offender and also what reinforces those values. This provides a clearer sense of your role and responsibilities. From an MI perspective, a single person working with an offender is not responsible for enforcing change, but instead for finding and fostering the intrinsic motivation that will be necessary to facilitate change.

MI, as a change-focused interaction, places the responsibility for behavior change on the offender. It is exhausting to try to convince a person to do something that he or she doesn't choose to do. Woefully, many who work with offenders feel that sense of exhaustion, another reason for the spread of MI in offender service agencies—using MI brings energy and renewal into your daily work. When MI is done skillfully, it is the offender who voices the arguments for change. How can that be? How do you do this? The first step is to establish an empathic and collaborative relationship (to be discussed at greater length in Chapters 2 and 5). A second step is to watch and listen for the person's values, and to explore how his or her current behavior fits within the context of these deeply held values. Discrepancy (the subject of Chapter 7) exists when there is a gap, or disconnect, between values and actions. MI draws attention to the idea that discrepancy underlies the perceived importance of change. No discrepancy means no motivation. Discrepancy amplifies *the offender's own reasons for change.* Highlighting this discrepancy creates an appetite for change. Once again, MI places you in the position of guiding an offender toward change rather than forcing or taking responsibility for the process.

5. *MI suggests effective ways of handling resistance and can keep difficult situations from getting worse.* Motivation is not a fixed characteristic, like adult height or having brown eyes. Instead, it is a condition or state, and it can be enhanced or diminished by the approach one chooses to take when working with the offender. Some professionals have been taught to break through the offender's denial, rationalization, or excuses by being direct and confrontational: "You've got a problem. You have to change. You'd better change or else!" However, many studies find that this confrontational counseling style limits effectiveness (e.g., Hubble, Duncan, & Miller, 1999; Miller & Rollnick, 2003). One early study of counseling style in alcohol treatment found that a directive–confrontational style produced twice the resistance and only half as many "positive" client behaviors as did a supportive, client-centered approach (Miller, Benefield, & Tonigan, 1993). The more the counselor confronted the problem behavior, the more the clients drank at 12-month follow-up. Thus, not only is a confrontational style less effective, but it can actually make matters worse. Still, many in direct service positions (e.g., probation or parole officers, correctional staff) or administration would object to the idea that there is a need to develop a supportive counseling style. After all, not everyone is a counselor, and we all play different roles within offender systems. Still, it is important for even noncounseling staff persons who interact with offenders to get back into the game of behavior change. Everyone works together to facilitate offender rehabilitation and reentry.

Instead of using a confrontational approach, some turn to a logical approach, employing advice or reasoning: "Why don't you just . . . ?" "Do you know what this behavior is doing to you?" "Here's how you should go about this . . . ." However, while not as directly challenging to the client's beliefs or behaviors as the confrontational approach, approaching the offender with logic or reason can be equally problematic. Just as with confrontational approaches, a logical or advice-giving stance can come across as patronizing, authoritarian, or forceful. Further, it is likely that the person has already considered these possibilities and may have reasons for not following such advice. Once again, we find that a more supportive and client-centered style may be the key to enhancing motivation.

These negative interaction styles are likely to decrease motivation, and may in turn worsen behavioral problems. When these methods fail, we often respond by pushing harder, only to find that the offender pushes back. In other words, when you escalate with confrontation or logical reasoning, the offender escalates as well, firmly defending an entrenched position. This further consolidates a commitment to the status quo.

"You've got a problem."   ⟶ "No, I don't."

"Why don't you . . . ?"   ⟶ "That won't work for me."

"You'd better change or else!" ⟶ "Take your best shot!"

This is clearly not the goal. You don't want to create a situation where the offender only defends the "don't change" side of the equation. Instead, you want to create an environment in which you and the offender can discuss both sides but also foster the growth of commitment to change. Decreasing resistance, or at the least not responding to resistance with direct confrontation and debate, is part of that. MI provides the framework and the tools through which we can have more productive and positive conversations about change.

WHERE WE GO FROM HERE

In this text, you will learn about the use of MI for offender rehabilitation and reentry. In Chapters 1–10, we emphasize the core philosophy of MI, as well as useful tools and strategies for engaging and understanding the offender. In Chapters 11–12 we discuss building a bridge to change, or how we focus on important goals, encourage change talk, and build upon the offender's strengths to promote meaningful and lasting change. And finally, in Chapters 13–15 we describe MI in practice in offender service systems, which involves promoting a culture of change, implementation science, and the flexibility of MI in different agencies and systems. Throughout, we use a combination of descriptive language, or language that tells you *what* to do, and injunctive language, which tells you *how* to do it. We also provide examples and anecdotes from practitioners across the globe with experience in implementing MI in diverse settings. We hope you find this text, and this approach, beneficial as you begin your own journey in using MI.

CHAPTER 2

THE SPIRIT OF MOTIVATIONAL INTERVIEWING

> My humanity is bound up in yours, for we can
> only be human together.
>   —DESMOND TUTU

MI is, first and foremost, a way of *being* with people. It is not therapy. It is not a list of techniques or strategies to make people change, or to make them want to change. Nor is it a friendship, or a way of disarming someone with a friendly smile and warm manner that communicates naiveté while maintaining an undercurrent of reasoned purpose. Instead, MI is a way of allowing you to be yourself, and to form a relationship with another person that fosters continued motivation, respect, and meaningful change.

As introduced in Chapter 1, traditional offender systems have emphasized the importance of superficial compliance, though more modern thought recognizes that the true goal is lasting behavior change. Much of the training in criminal justice and corrections stresses the technique over the principle. Officer safety, electronic monitoring, the process of custody, and victim issues are topics well known and prevalent in the field. Such training is presented in step-by-step fashion, focusing on *how* to do it. The *why* is assumed and often goes unquestioned. Methods of treatment and rehabilitation have followed the same pattern in that we emphasize how to initiate treatment, how to ensure treatment compliance, or how to do the basics of offender counseling. But *why* we do these things has been deemphasized.

This overemphasis on techniques affects the practice of MI with offenders. Often we focus on the *how,* believing MI is a series of techniques that can be used to persuade offenders to follow the rules and participate in treatment. However, such a narrow focus barely breaches the surface of what must be deeper work. Instead, you should think about the combined heart, mind, and skills that capture the essential spirit of MI; these skills are necessary to shift your work toward the business of behavior change (Clark, 2005). It is something you develop in your way of being that fosters your work *with* rather than *on* a person. Thus, offenders are not passive or even resistant recipients of your medicine or advice, but rather active participants who co-create new lives. Further, they deserve respect and understanding, as they best understand themselves and their own capacities for change.

This chapter examines four interconnected elements of the spirit of MI: partnership, acceptance, compassion, and evocation. These four elements form the acronym PACE—and they most certainly help you keep *pace* with an offender. They underscore the necessary beliefs and behaviors that facilitate success in offender rehabilitation and reentry. Please note, though, that to begin the practice of MI, one does not have to be an expert in all aspects of PACE. Rather, learning is a process, and you gain competency over time and through effort. New efforts become experience, experience becomes habit, and eventually habit becomes practice. Let us now discuss this spirit of MI that will become our practice.

PARTNERSHIP

In Chapter 1, we differentiated compliance from true behavior change. When you seek only compliance, or to stabilize and control that which we deem out of control, then the task is clear. You decide what you want and find the right mix of power and authority to obtain acquiescence. This creates a typical "us versus them" relationship. But if you seek meaningful behavior change, you need your clients as allies rather than opponents. The task is to develop a partnership, or collaboration.

> *If you seek meaningful behavior change, you need your clients as allies rather than opponents.*

Partnership is the first of the four elements forming the spirit of

MI. Partnership assumes the presence and participation of more than one person in the relationship. Your values are important, as are those of the person with whom you are working. Persons being supervised come to us because the courts have ordered it so—whether for incarceration, community supervision, or mandated treatment. An important nuance in the spirit of MI is that one works with offenders to change the behavior that led to punishment; you do not work with them to inflict further punishment.

Why this collaboration? Because all change is self-change. The person is the real agent of change. No staff member or counselor can know people better than they know themselves. Just as none of us are the same, all offenders are unique and different as well. Our purpose is to be curious. You should listen to the person in front of you, find out what your clients think, how they understand the world around them, what or who they value, and how their emotions and experiences have built their beliefs and expectations. In MI, the person takes center stage. But why? Because you alone cannot make someone change, or make people different from who they are. Change is driven by individual motivation—not information or advice. Fostering motivation requires knowledge that augments your own. Such knowledge comes from the client. Partnering with the client ensures activation and involvement in the change process, which may be one of the most critical pieces of achieving positive client outcomes (Duncan, Miller, Wampold, & Hubble, 2009). In short, connect rather than calculate. It is less about planning or strategizing than about other aspects of your work. While guidance and influence remain important, willingness and participation from the client count perhaps more. See an example of this in Box 2.1, in which a new client struggles with these issues.

The need for partnership can be problematic for corrections and criminal justice. Some view a partnership with the client as discretionary, or contingent on the offender's behavior. In practice, this discretionary or contingent relationship means that you develop a partnership with the agreeable people who follow the rules, but you suspend that idea of partnership for persons who break the rules, or who prove difficult to work with. Assuming this position detaches you from the change process and puts you in the position of an observer, passively reacting to what the client does. Instead, partnership is an active process, with important roles for both persons involved in the relationship.

The MI spirit of partnership also suspends the acts of telling, teaching, or advice giving. While these behaviors certainly have a place in work with offender clients, they may be more coercive than conducive

---

BOX 2.1. PARTNERSHIP

Mark had a lengthy history of drug-related and violent offending. He was required to see me, and after having asked around about me, was unhappy to learn I had also worked in probation. He was aggravated in the waiting room before our initial visit, and was even careful to move his chair several feet farther away from me when we met. He immediately began: "I know you were a PO, and as far as I'm concerned, you're all one big gang. You all stick up for each other. I don't see how we can ever work together."

"Ah. You're worried that I've already judged you," I said. He stared, and I added, "I'm glad you brought it up right away. You don't like to waste time. We should be able to make some progress if you decide to give me a chance."

"I'm not saying I will," he said.

"Okay. Totally up to you. But let's say you do decide to try. Any ideas about how I can work with you so we can be successful?"

Mark thought for a moment. "The only guy who ever helped me made a point of not making me feel ashamed. If I fell off of the horse, he helped me get back on without wasting time asking why I was stupid enough to fall off in the first place."

"You want help getting back on track for the future, not talking about past problems. That works for me. What else?"

"He didn't make me sit in a chair for an hour, talking about stuff."

I nodded. "It doesn't help you to sit and talk about problems for an hour straight. We'll need to break things up a bit." Mark agreed to give it a try, and we worked together for over a year.

—Rob Axsen, Pacific Community Resources Society, British Columbia, Canada

---

to change, and they only emphasize the control one has over the other person. Unfortunately, traditional corrections and criminal justice practices have valued being in control of a person over building a bridge to promote progress and change. The problem, however, with establishing control and giving advice is that you risk becoming so central to the process that you no longer acknowledge or seek the client's own capacity for change. (This is called the "expert trap" and will be discussed further in Chapter 4.) When you are filled with advice and expertise—no matter how accurate or well-meaning it may be—you are like a full balloon, lacking handles or edges that allow your client to grab hold. And if one assumes that the client is similarly full of expertise, it becomes like trying to attach two inflated balloons together—impossible. One should avoid a singular focus on a preconceived agenda and instead follow and respond to the client in the moment.

But within this is another challenge. What about responsibilities to the court, to society, or other important correctional or criminal justice system goals? It is possible to suspend the role of authority, primarily in one's interactional style, in order to establish this critical partnership. Suspend, but not eliminate. As agents of the court, staff members within an organization or facility, or specialists working with mandated clients, you must be both aware of and honest with offender clients. Being in partnership does not mean denying your role, or values, or your goals in preventing further illegal behavior. Partnership necessitates genuineness. You can suspend an authoritarian persona in order to develop a true collaboration for change, but you cannot push aside your responsibility for reporting problematic behavior, or the reality that problem behavior may carry sanctions. It is a careful balance that we will continue to examine throughout this text.

Partnership is difficult. As with the other key aspects of the spirit of MI, partnership is fluid and also delicate. It may run counter to what agents in offender systems have been taught as the "right" way to work with offenders. Yet understand that you cannot do it alone, and that you need the offender on this journey toward change. Partnering also requires a change in heart-set toward a nonwavering respect for those with whom you work. We seek an alliance that moves beyond a focus on requirements and compliance, and one that will bring about lasting and meaningful change.

ACCEPTANCE

Acceptance is a way of being with people that is critical in the development of partnership, and in the use of MI. It permeates the literature on motivating meaningful change. And it represents an interesting paradox—you want the person to change, yet accepting the person for who he or she is facilitates the change process. Acceptance includes all that the offender brings in with them, including a history of illegal or other problem behavior, excuses, failures within the system, and the like. This acceptance of what has already happened does not imply that you would condone the behavior or excuse harm, but merely that you acknowledge it as a reality. You cannot change what has already been. You can only work to change what could be.

Acceptance as a respectful stance has an extensive history in offender research. Bonta et al. (2008) appealed for correctional staff members to "establish a positive, warm and respectful relationship with the client" (p. 262) in order to influence change. Acceptance, however, is much more than just a respectful stance, and is certainly not a simple task. Hostility, violence, deceit, and other factors can interfere with our own willingness to accept. How do you foster acceptance within a client relationship? Four key components of acceptance are crucial: absolute worth, accurate empathy, autonomy, and affirmation.

Absolute Worth

The first aspect of acceptance involves an attitude that every person has worth and potential. MI represents a dramatic departure from conventional justice work. Nowhere is this more apparent than the call to accept the inherent worth of every offender. The challenge is to look within and decide whether or not criminal behavior negates a person's humanity. To us, it does not. Every person has worth and should be accorded basic human respect.

This is personal. You must decide if wrongful acts make a person less human. In spite of their crimes, are offenders still worth helping? Those who embrace the spirit of MI would readily agree that they are. Yet this sensible and humane stance is often overshadowed by decades of emotionally driven rhetoric which says that offenders are fundamentally different than other people. Provocative descriptions of crime and criminals, often meant to invoke fear and revulsion, demonize offenders as persons who are different from responsible, law-abiding citizens (e.g., Samenow, 1978; Yochelson & Samenow, 1977). Such views do not lend themselves to developing compassion, respect, or interest in a person's basic humanity, but instead lead to a punitive indifference that may only perpetuate the problem.

The opposite of absolute worth is judgmental condemnation, which has already played a major role in offenders' lives. They have been judged worthy or not by virtue of their own behavior. Offender systems are predicated on judgment, and one is implicitly made to feel "right" by correcting the mistakes or misbehavior of those who were "wrong." Although it may be human nature to judge, it is integral to the development of genuine relationships to foster acceptance. A climate for change is enhanced when a person feels valued, respected, and treated as a whole person, or more than simply his or her past. See an example of this in Box 2.2, where we highlight the idea that sincerely valuing another person is an important precursor to change.

BOX 2.2. ABSOLUTE WORTH

A couple of years ago I was working as a researcher in Stockholm. A PO had asked me to use a brief motivational interviewing program with one of her clients. Hanna was a 30-year-old heroin user, and like many clients, she was highly defensive, expecting to hear a lengthy list of flaws in her personality and problems with her behavior. Instead, I began our conversation with "Hanna, how nice to see you. You look like a typical Swedish young woman to me. And in your summer dress, you look like you just came from a day out. I am really looking forward to working with you, but before we begin, I would like to know a little more about you—what you're interested in, your hobbies, the kinds of music you like, and what makes you feel good about yourself. Please, begin."

Hanna looked surprised, perhaps wondering if I was really a part of the correctional staff. She then told me many things. She enjoyed playing the guitar and found herself to be quite skilled at it. She had once before owned her own business, and she liked doing nails and other cosmetics. She had a 10-year-old son currently living with her mother, and she wanted to be better at taking care of him. Hanna gave me a lot of material about her life, her hopes, and her future goals.

I summarized our conversation: "You understand and love music. You know how to run a business, and that involves some pretty advanced skills. Your son is a great love in your life, and he is very important to you." It only took a few minutes to show her that I valued her as a person. And after what could have been a quite difficult and defensive conversation, she instead saw that I could view her as more than just her drug problem.

—Carl Ake Farbring, MSc, *Swedish Prison and Probation Administration,*
2000–2010, Akersberga, Sweden

Accurate Empathy

A second aspect of acceptance is accurate empathy, a form of focused interest that breeds openness and understanding toward another person. In the spirit of MI and acceptance, you don't listen to offenders to collect their conversations as evidence of their criminal thinking and behavior, to be used against them or to coerce them into agreeing that they need help. You listen to truly understand the world as they see it. In this new climate of assisting behavior change, accurate empathy is critical. You listen to people the way we want to be listened to. Carl Rogers described empathy as "to sense the client's inner world of private personal meanings as if it were our own, but without ever losing the 'as if' quality"

(Rogers, 1957, p. 99). In other words, we must focus on the other person's world as he or she sees it, rather than trying to interpret it as we see it.

Empathy is a powerful force that can topple assumptions about clients and bring you closer to seeing things as they do. But what is accurate empathy, really? You may rely on sympathy or pity to presume you understand. You may use reassurances or tell your own stories to convey the idea that you've been there too, that you know what it feels like. Kindness and camaraderie may be helpful, but they're also *not empathy*. Empathy is a true act of the heart—an effort to "learn" the person, and to listen closely and with curiosity to know their inner world of meaning. Imagine yourself visiting an alien world—your client's world—where you rely on nothing more than the client and your own senses to ground yourself and to navigate your surroundings (Bohart & Tallman, 1999). With no frame of reference of your own, you must take the client's views and beliefs at face value and interpret everything through the client's frame. This is accurate empathy, or the point at which you let go of your own contexts and presumptions and try to truly understand another person's world.

Autonomy–Support

Another element of acceptance is autonomy–support. We have already noted that the spirit of MI calls us to extend dignity and respect to people under supervision. With this also comes the right of choice, or a person's freedom to choose his or her own course of action. Autonomy is the individual's perception of him- or herself as the determining agent of an action (i.e., "I choose to do this"). A person will work harder and make more lasting change when he or she makes a choice to do so. Thus, autonomy–support is critical in the change process. A person must make a reasoned choice about change, and our role involves not only facilitating change, but also supporting autonomy. Acceptance assumes autonomy, in that one must value a person's right to choose as part of accepting him or her as a person of worth.

A clear problem, however, is that many offender systems are structured in such a way as to deemphasize autonomous choice. Much of the work in these systems is about control and eliciting compliance, and the assumed role is to *make* someone change. The reality is that one is never capable of *making* a person do anything. You set the climate for behavior change when you shift your view of client decision making. A probation officer who tells his or her client, "You can't leave the jurisdiction" is not stating the literal truth (Miller & Rollnick, 2013). The client is perhaps fully capable of leaving the area. Instead, what the probation officer means is that there are consequences for behaviors that violate court orders. It is the same when you tell a client, "You can't drink," or "You must attend counseling." What this really means is that you want them to make responsible choices about drinking or attending treatment, but the freedom to choose always remains with the client.

Acknowledging autonomy requires us to relinquish power that we never had in the first place. We cannot take away the person's right to choose. That belongs to him or her. Recognizing and honoring this ultimately leads to more effective and lasting change, as coercion fosters a sense of being manipulated and therefore undermines internal motivation (Walters et al., 2007). Too much pushing can make a person less likely to change (Miller & Rollnick, 2013). Though the consequences of not changing are perhaps more obvious and to us, more important, we can build autonomy by listing consequences in a neutral way and emphasizing personal choice, as described by one of our colleagues in Box 2.3.

BOX 2.3. AUTONOMY–SUPPORT

Sean was a court-mandated client who greeted me in the waiting room with an expression of undisguised distaste. I had not yet finished closing the door to my office when he said, "Look, nothing against you, but this is all crap. I don't need to be here. Just one more thing costing me money I don't have."

"You're really frustrated with all the hoops you have to jump through," I reflected. His face changed from angry to fatigued. He said he had been handling his own problems all his life, and that he didn't need me. "I understand," I told him. "It's not my job to make you do anything you don't want to do. If you want to cancel today, there won't be any charge."

"I can't do that," he said. "That means jail again. No way."

"Coming here would at least help you stay out of jail," I noted.

"I guess."

"Okay," I responded. "How would you feel about going through with our interview today to see if we can find other ways to make this work out for you? The court says you have to be here, but they don't tell us what we have to talk about. That's up to you."

"I can do that," Sean said. He sighed. "Sorry about before. Since the DUI, it feels like everybody has a piece of me . . . telling me what to do, you know?"

I thought for a minute. "Maybe we can find a way to help you feel more confident that nothing like that will happen to you again."

"That'd be good," he said ruefully. "Actually, this is my second DUI, and I didn't think it ever *would* happen again, but here I am."

Now we had something to talk about.

—*Ron Skidmore, MA, LPC, Third Coast Counseling Center, Grand Rapids, Michigan*

Affirmation

Finally, the last piece of acceptance is affirmation. Verbalize your support of clients. Affirm and validate their survival—they've been through adversity, survived it, and may still struggle to keep going. Compliment them on the decision to keep trying. This requires you to use accurate empathy, so that your affirmations are genuine and respect their will and effort. This affirms their worth. To offer such compliments or affirmations is not softhearted or used only to convey kindness, but purposefully creates a climate for change. Affirmation helps create a safe atmosphere that communicates partnership and support. It also promotes trust. Trust is a key element of acceptance. But most importantly, affirmations mobilize clients' strengths, including their past successes, talents, knowledge, capacities, and resources. This is exemplified in Box 2.4. One must carefully and relentlessly affirm what they are capable of, as they may come from a place of harsh judgment by others or self-criticism to the point that they no longer know what their strengths are.

Those who work with offenders may worry that focusing on the positives, or affirming the person's worth and abilities, disregards the person's past illegal behaviors. But affirmation is far more than just being positive and complimentary. Affirmation acknowledges a simple truth: People change through their distinctive abilities and attributes, rather than their failures or deficits. As social beings, we seek the approval of others. Here, the goal is to approve that which makes people capable of fostering their own self-change.

When we examine these four conditions, the idea of acceptance begins to take defined shape. Regardless of the crime he or she has committed, each person has *worth* and potential as human being. Since all change is self-change, *accurate empathy* allows understanding of the other person's perspective. We recognize the offender's *autonomy* to choose what must be done. And we *affirm* his or her resources and efforts. These four elements promote a climate of change. Acceptance is not a private experience or a quiet commitment to certain feelings or values, but something purposeful that is communicated through your words and actions.

COMPASSION

Approaches for effective offender rehabilitation and reentry involve specific methods and skills. The practice of MI is no different. Here we

---

BOX 2.4. AFFIRMATION

Our clients seldom hear affirmations, especially outside of our own contacts with them. Our clients' worlds are sometimes difficult and cruel places. As a probation officer, I focus on affirming effort and achievement. Things I say to do this include:

- "Nice work filling out those six job applications today!"
- "You look sharp."
- "You gave him some honest feedback."
- "Group is for you—this is a safe place for you to bring up those kinds of issues."
- "I appreciate your honesty."
- "You've worked hard to pay off those fines."

Lamonte had recently been diagnosed with diabetes and lost 20 pounds between appointments. It was noticeable. When I said, "Lamonte, you look great!" a huge smile came over his face, and you could see him sit up straighter, already more confident. He told me that he had done it by not eating treats, cake, or ice cream every night like he had before. I responded with, "You're making big strides, and it shows." He was excited to share how he changed his eating habits.

Anthony had spent 4 months seeking a job but with no success. His spirits were down. I told him, "If you keep at it, it will happen." He was discouraged. I shared with him the list of places that were hiring and expressed faith in his efforts to keep going. Three days later, Anthony called to tell me he had an interview. "Awesome! I knew it would happen for you," I replied.

—Todd Roberts, Sixth Judicial District, Iowa Department of Corrections, Cedar Rapids, Iowa

---

have begun to describe a spirit and attitude that must be learned and practiced over time. These encompass the mind-set and skill set of MI. But there is also a heart-set, which is nowhere more apparent than with *compassion*.

Compassion takes deliberate intention. It does not come easily, and it may at times feel counterintuitive. You work to promote the client's welfare and to give priority to his or her needs while still maintaining reasonable focus on the demands of your own job and values. If the only goal was compliance, then simply anesthetizing all your clients would accomplish that. Administering an anesthetic would simply *stop* any behavior that is unacceptable, frustrating, or noncompliant, and would do so in a humane and equal way. But that is not the goal. It might be easier if your clients were safe, asleep, and thus unable to challenge your perceptions of what is "right," but the true goal is behavior change. This involves a deliberate commitment to pursue the best interests and welfare of another, thus naturally initiating a process that requires partnership, acceptance, and compassion.

In Chapter 1, we noted common views and perceptions of offenders permeating society. Few feel genuine compassion toward those who have committed crimes and hurt others. A call for compassion would result in a predictable rallying cry: "They don't deserve it!" Such an attitude is evident from our laws and history of treating and managing offenders in our prisons and communities. It is perhaps all too easy to fall into this trap. We work with difficult people. We face multiple and sometimes conflicting demands. After a long, particularly difficult day, or a disheartening outcome with a specific client, it is natural to blame people for their faults and lose sight of their humanity and struggle. But the spirit of MI does not include judgment of who is most worthy or deserving of consideration. Viewing a person as bad, and therefore undeserving of forgiveness or a chance at a new life, is simply incompatible with a motivational style.

Enter the spirit of compassion. Compassion takes root in varying religious, spiritual, and philosophical schools of thought. For example, Hindu definitions of compassion denote two forms: compassion for persons who suffer but have committed no wrong, and compassion for those who suffer because they have committed wrong (Balslev & Evers, 2009; Gandhi, 1978). Buddhism conceptualizes an act of compassion as one that frees someone from suffering (Dalai Lama & Vreeland, 2001; Nhat Hanh, 1999; Salzberg, 1995). Islamic faith describes the interconnectedness and shared emotion of humanity as reflective of God, invoking strong images of compassion for fellow humans (Balslev & Evers, 2009). And Christianity characterizes compassion as a method of communicating love or forgiveness (Armstrong, 2010; Miller, 2000). So what is compassion, as we consider our own work with offenders? It isn't merely empathy in response to another's suffering, but also attention to values, patience, and connection with another's human frailty. Compassion requires both courage and vulnerability.

MI teaches that a change of heart cannot be imposed; it can only be chosen. Why? Because a change of heart comes from one's beliefs, values, and desires. One of the most powerful human motivators is the power of the committed heart. This commitment of heart involves more than one person, as it is not just the client but also we who have values, beliefs, and desires that move us in the direction of change. This component of the spirit of MI insists upon meeting on a common, heartfelt ground. If you hesitate at the thought of fully and unabashedly embracing compassion as a practice with offenders, you are not alone. Compassion toward offenders presents a unique opportunity. You must challenge your own preconceived notions of what a person values, and access his or her world of values with acceptance and accurate empathy. In this effort, you can ill afford to remain aloof and distant, still expecting to engage fully.

Even from a place of compassion, it may be difficult to see how some offenders are capable of change, given their challenges and lack of resources. This stems from the biased nature of the population sampled. Those you see day to day are having problems, and many of them are experiencing severe problems.

> *MI teaches that a change of heart cannot be imposed; it can only be chosen.*

How can you maintain both compassion and hope for offenders who additionally face poverty, mental illness, physical disability, histories of trauma and maltreatment, little education, unstable housing, daily exposure to violence, poor social support, and the like? You see them at their worst, or when they are only just beginning their recovery from their lowest point. Pity is all too easily mistaken for compassion, yet lapsing into hopelessness makes you less effective at facilitating change.

There is a price for pessimism. One of the largest studies of probation in the United Kingdom found that though a majority of defendants were successful in overcoming obstacles and earned release from court jurisdiction, their supervising officers were "three times more likely to report that their probationer would *not* be able to stop offending than the probationers themselves" (Farrall, 2002). Of greater concern is that as probationers' involvement with criminal justice supervision increased, the less they believed themselves capable of desisting from criminal behavior. In other words, the more they see staff in offender agencies, the less they think they can be helped. We must commit to reversing these trends. But how to do it? MI and working with compassion help maintain humor, hope, and gratitude. They keep us from taking ourselves too seriously. The tremendous will of the human spirit is more easily revealed in the addict with a fierce hold on early sobriety, or the single mother who resolves to do her best to guarantee safety for her child, than in examining only those who have never known adversity. We are inspired and privileged when people share their intimate pain, raw humanness, and resilience.

EVOCATION

Evocation is the fourth and final element of the spirit of MI and represents as dramatic a departure from traditional offender work as partnership, acceptance, and compassion. The mind-set for evocation aligns with strengths-based approaches in that you trust that people already have within them what is needed for positive change. The goal is to help them activate it. MI calls you to draw forth their aspirations, values, and competencies, or that which makes them distinctly and individually human. Berg (1994) cautions us to stay close to the client's definition of the problem and possible solutions, since it is the client rather than us who must make proscribed changes. Most reentry and remediation plans are born from our perspectives, but this does not make sense. The plan isn't ours; it belongs to someone else. This is a source of so much frustration in offender work. We view ourselves rather than the clients as the focus of services, and when they don't complete a plan we've devised, we view it as their failure rather than our own.

Evocation arises naturally from ambivalence, a concept described further in Chapter 7. Offenders already have within them arguments both for and against change. A part of them does want to change. A naturally or learned evocative style can elicit their capacities that support the part of them that wants to change. In Chapters 9 and 10 we will further examine evocation as a practice and the role of ambivalence as a precursor to the change you seek. For now, it's important to realize the upside to patience and waiting for strengths to emerge: you only need wait for clients to discover that which is within them, and they will be more committed to exploring strengths than lamenting weaknesses. This will guide them toward more lasting and natural change. The spirit of evocation urges you to elicit and encourage motivations that already exist.

Our field is held hostage by the deficit model (Clark, 1995). There is a core belief that offenders come to us deficient: they lack skills, they lack insight, and their values are somehow askew. The proof is in their behavior—*just look at what they've done.* Surely they are the ones with the "problems." Their criminal behavior is symptomatic of a deeper problem. The field as a whole has held the position that if we can iden- tify the problem, we can find a solution. We then search for current faults and past failures within the individual and his or her environment, attending primarily to the offender's defects and deficits. This search is sequential: find and recognize the problem (assessment), work to under- stand the problem (diagnosis), and determine the level of service needed (risk) before taking action (treatment). You expect that the offender will agree with our diagnosis and solution (compliance) and hope that the offender will understand the problem as you do (insight). The real prob- lem, however, is that we typically do this without true collaboration or understanding of the offender. We do ask for input, but only so that we can complete the sequence in the way we think is most helpful. Less credence is given to the offender's understanding and definition of the problem if it differs from ours, and we formulate a plan that relies on his or her acquiescence rather than evocation.

Evocation requires a focus on strengths. You communicate that "You have what you need, and together we will find it." Problems do have an impact, just as risk and diagnostic assessments have their place in what you do. But evocation aligns us with promise and possibility, drawing our attention to what clients naturally possess. Evocation is about capacity rather than deficit. You turn your attention to what someone could do, rather than what he or she hasn't done, or has failed to do. For example, in Box 2.5 (on page 30) we see a brief demonstration of how evocation can be so powerful in not only engaging the client but also in facilitating the spirit that is essential to our work.

By focusing on strengths, allowing natural ambivalence to surface, and exploring that in a genuine, compassionate, and collaborative way, one can begin to facilitate true behavior change. You need only listen and know where to start.

BOX 2.5. EVOCATION

When I first began working as an alcohol and drug counselor, I was the director of four women's recovery homes. Several of the women in these homes came to us through the legal system. Once during a nightly group session, we were discussing strengths. The women were having a difficult time coming up with any strengths, particularly related to job skills they might use to obtain employment to support their families. To one, I said, "You were a drug dealer. Were you any good?"

She seemed surprised. She answered, "Yeah, I made some good money."

"Good," I said. "That means you were a good salesperson. Now how about the metric system? Anybody learn about that from dealing?" And on we went. I have to admit that I couldn't believe what was coming out, and I'm sure they were surprised, too. By the end of the group, they had laughed, cried, and shared more of themselves than I'd ever heard from them before. I think we bonded over that conversation, unconventional though it was. It wasn't just about their deficits. And the women left feeling hopeful, strong, and that better lives were possible. That's got to be a good thing.

—DeeDee Stout, MA, CADC-II, California State University,
Monterey Bay, Emeryville, California

CHAPTER 3

THE ART OF LISTENING

The more you know, the less you understand.
—LAO TZU

The ability to listen is the foundation of MI. Deep listening is basic to engaging, focusing, eliciting, and planning, the four processes that are at the core of MI, and underlies our communication with the client throughout. There are some occasions, such as serving probation orders or taking someone into custody, that naturally call for a directive style. Yet listening can aid even the toughest of criminal justice tasks. Many situations present an opportunity to guide and influence long-term behavior change, calling for a client-centered style that emphasizes listening. In this chapter, we will describe and demonstrate the skill of deep listening and provide examples that highlight the importance of listening in working with offenders from an MI perspective. We will also introduce reflective listening, a necessary skill for engaging the client (see Chapters 5 and 6), but also used throughout conversations about change.

WHY LISTEN?

We do not know why people choose to change. For each person, it is an individual decision, driven by unique values, goals, and desires. In order to understand someone and learn what may help him or her achieve these goals, listening becomes necessary. This is more complicated with offenders. In another setting, with a different population, you would be in a better position to take the person at face value, your perceptions

31

free from the taint of prior knowledge. But for offenders, a judge or jury has already made a determination of guilt. Records describe what the offender has already done or said. You may have personal experience with an individual through his or her prior contacts with the system. Your expectations are set. As a result, it becomes difficult to fully and openly listen. You listen for what you want to hear, or what you "should" hear, and judge the person's behavior as good or bad. But is it truly necessary to re-create what has already happened? Instead, perhaps it is better to experience clients as they are in the moment, without placing them in a moral category or seeking to confirm preexisting judgments.

Some aspects of our work have clear answers—they are either right, or they are wrong. In arithmetic, an equation can be right or wrong. When you approach a traffic light and it has turned red, you stop. You do not have to be open-minded about something as absolute as a red light at an intersection. Yet in working with offenders, such certainty is scarce. When we work with people to influence change, we rarely have the answers. Such work requires an open mind, and we open our minds through *listening*.

Have you ever been given puzzle pieces but no box? It is not an easy task to fit the pieces together without the aid of the completed picture from the box-top to guide you. But if you were to attempt this task, you would find yourself far more attentive to each individual piece, acutely aware of its colors and contour, and less quick to judge its role in the larger picture. This is comparable to how you should use MI to approach offenders. Without a picture, you are more likely to listen intently and with curiosity, taking each piece at face value, letting yourself learn and be intrigued by how people are put together. Ironically, one of the biggest barriers to deep listening is your own experience and training. Experience leads to assumptions about the offender's problem, limiting one's openness to hearing what he or she has to say.

WHERE TO START?

In Chapter 2, we discussed the need for accurate empathy. Developing this empathy requires listening. A good listener is a witness—listening with curious interest, absorbing as much as possible. You listen to discover and appreciate the uniqueness of the person, seeing him or her as more than just another offender, a category of risk, or a mental health diagnosis. You avoid listening with filters, or selecting only the evidence that substantiates your preconceived judgments. You work to suspend your beliefs and to be impartial, even when you have a strong interest in the outcome. Giving up your own sense of importance and expertise is an important first step, as are preparation, planful silence, and of course, practice.

Prepare Your Mind

Deep listening will not come easily to an unprepared mind. For a moment, consider the practice of meditation. Meditation is not something one would typically associate with the world of offender management and treatment, though increasing evidence supports the use of mindfulness and other meditation-based practices in improving mental health (e.g., Grossman, Niemann, Schmidt, & Walach, 2004; Mace, 2007; Shapiro & Carlson, 2009). Nor do we often think of meditation as a tool to help us listen—after all, isn't meditation supposed to be silent? But in practice, traditions like meditation, mindfulness, and yoga teach us to work toward focusing the mind and identifying and noticing judgments, reactions, or attachments to strongly held beliefs. MI and the practice of deep listening have us do the same in that we observe and set aside our judgments of the person and his or her situation, as well as our attachment to the idea that we are experts who can singlehandedly fix the problem.

Stop Talking

We, as professionals, talk too much. Though it may sound humorous, we do not say this lightly or frivolously. In our society, talking is the norm, and we are praised for speaking our minds. Instead, Camp (2002) posits that "Not talking is hard. We're trained through education to know all the answers and to blurt them out at the first opportunity. We have been rewarded time and time again for knowing the correct answer. Our life has revolved around our intelligence. We go to great pains to let people know what we know" (p. 153). Talking is expected. Talking demonstrates your expertise, experience, and insight into others' problems. This is perhaps nowhere more true than for those who work with offenders. The work carries its own unique burden—the requirement that you must know all of the answers and, through your own knowledge and experience, make right the offenders' wrongs. In MI this is called the expert trap (discussed further in Chapter 4), the tendency to present ourselves as experts who have the solution to the offender's dilemma, which triggers our urge to talk. Avoiding this trap involves letting go

It is through listening that you can initiate meaningful conversation and change.

of your assumptions of "rightness," or the expectation that you should give advice. Other reasons for excessive talking include training, the desire to be right, or discomfort with silence or ambiguity. Because of these, we find ourselves unable to stop talking, which prevents good listening. And even when we do stop talking, it is to think of what to say next rather than to listen. Yet it is through listening that you learn about the other person and can initiate meaningful conversation and change.

Practice, Practice, Practice

A third component of effective listening is practice. Unfortunately, it is easy to reason your way out of this necessary effort, making an assumption that you already know how to listen. Listening is something you have done your whole life, right? While it is true that we all know what it means to listen and have experience doing so, it's still difficult to listen effectively. Listening is an acquired skill, much like learning how to play the piano or tennis. Without practice, you remain a novice. This chapter emphasizes "professional listening," which requires practice. Why practice something that seems so straightforward? Because it's easy to listen to the surface information garnered through unskilled listening, though staying at this superficial level of understanding neglects necessary information about the offenders' internal dilemmas, values, and experiences that drive personal motivation for change. The four processes of MI—engagement, focusing, evocation, and planning—all involve continued listening. MI inherently requires you to listen, and to practice your listening so that you can be most effective in facilitating change.

LISTENING BECOMES COMMUNICATION

Now you're prepared. Suppose you quietly listen to the client for a full 5 minutes. What does this look like? If you presume "quiet" listening means remaining motionless, like a mannequin in a store window, you will be passive and detached from the conversation, and the client will get nothing back and believe you aren't really listening. So while it is important to prepare the mind and offer quiet observation, it is equally important for the speaker to know you are listening. That is when listening becomes communication.

Even when we are silent, our nonverbal cues convey connection and understanding. Thomas Gordon (1970) called this "active listening," and doing this well is as important as anything you may say. Many readers are already aware of the nonverbal cues of listening, but it's worth reviewing them before we move on.

Undivided Attention

Giving undivided attention is not always easy in offender service environments. Common distractions include colleagues who stop by for a quick question or update, desk items like phones or pagers that ring, ping, or vibrate, or e-mail alerts on the computer that draw your attention away for time periods ranging from a few seconds to several minutes. Attention may also drift, consciously or unconsciously, and you may find yourself shuffling papers, taking notes, and checking the time. When these diversions dominate, the client is pushed aside. Such behaviors communicate disinterest and disrespect. Just because you *can* do two things at once does not mean you *should*—especially when listening. Explaining it away with "I'm busy" doesn't diminish the sense of superiority and self-importance conveyed to the client. Effective listening requires undivided attention. When it's time to listen, *just listen*. It's as simple as that.

Eye Contact

Eye contact expresses importance. A good listener maintains eye contact with the person who is speaking. A speaker's return eye contact may vacillate, with periodic glances away, particularly when remembering specific events or discussing delicate topics. We are mindful of vast cultural differences in this regard. Some cultures regard too much direct eye contact as disrespectful, while in other cultures, looking away while addressing someone is rude or insulting. Nevertheless, in most instances, eye contact communicates undivided attention. You will know the norms within your own culture, but remain sensitive to customs and interpersonal standards, especially when working with people of varying backgrounds. Consider, too, the norms involving seating position during a conversation. Place chairs too close together, and people feel uncomfortable. For some, chairs arranged so that the speaker and listener are directly facing one another makes it difficult to look away during the conversation. Setting chairs at an angle can make it easier for the speaker to break eye contact or to look at you when he or she wishes. Comfortable eye contact and personal space will encourage the speaker and facilitate greater communication in most contexts.

Facial Expressions

Facial expressions can communicate attention and understanding. One goal is for facial expression to mirror the speaker's content. In correctional settings, such content can range from boring and repetitive (e.g., "I've heard this too many times") to emotionally laden or personally disturbing. Some staff listeners choose to maintain a "poker face," or one that does not change in response to what the speaker says. They convince themselves that it's better to be objective or stay neutral when faced with such emotional talk from offenders, as that demonstrates a more professional or detached demeanor. However, a face with no expression offers little support to the speaker. Worse, in the absence of interpersonal feedback, many speakers will default to negative interpretations of what the listener is thinking. Limited visual feedback from your facial expression could generate anxiety in the speaker that you disapprove or are judging what they say.

In conversation, people often mirror each other's emotional expression. Sad expressions from the speaker prompt a sad face from the listener. Expressions of joy, fear, or surprise change the listener's facial expressions as well. Nonverbal mirroring of the client's emotions signals listening, understanding, and joining. An important exception, however, is client anger—rather than mirroring back anger, it is more appropriate to respond with expressions of concern and a calm demeanor.

REFLECTIVE LISTENING

Listening is important, but alone it just isn't enough. Speakers need to know that you have *heard* what they have said. Thus, you must reflect back to offenders the content of their statements, which may be more than simply the words they have said. Carl Rogers (1965) called this *accurate empathy,* which became a cornerstone of client-centered counseling.

Reflective listening is a skill. It communicates to the speaker that someone is listening, and that what they say is important and valuable. Rather than automatic conversational responses like nodding or saying, "uh huh," reflection requires that the listener focus on content and, just as with a visual reflection from a mirror, hold it up to the speaker for him or her to examine. Making a reflective statement engages our full attention, brings us into the conversation as active listeners, and provides feedback to the speaker about the listener's perception of what has been said. Let us consider the examples of reflective listening provided in Table 3.1.

While we cover reflective listening in more extensive detail in Chapter 6 during our discussion of engaging, a few points are worth noting here before we move on. First, when you reflect what the speaker has said, it is best to keep it simple. An important part of this is making a direct statement, which may be in contrast to what many have learned about reflective or other similar statements. Your prior training may emphasize introductory stems before the reflection, like "So what I hear you saying is . . . " or "So if I've got this right, what you're saying is . . . . " These phrases increase the amount that you're talking while not adding to the speaker's experience of being heard. The best reflections avoid such clutter and keep the conversation flowing by getting immediately to the point.

Second, remove "I" from reflective statements, since the point is really to reflect someone else rather than yourself. Prefacing reflections with phrases that draw attention to the listener is unnecessary and distracting. These include "So I heard you say . . . ," "What I hear you saying is . . . ," or "I believe what you're getting at is . . . . " Reflections are meant to show the person that you're trying to understand them. When you start with "I," it becomes about you, or communicates that the speaker is responsible for what you think. Instead, reflections should

TABLE 3.1. Examples of Reflective Listening

OFFENDER: I don't know how to cope. I mean, I get really stressed by my job, and I need a few drinks to calm down.

LISTENER: You use alcohol to deal with your stress.

OFFENDER: Look at my life—look at where I live and the part of town I'm in. Given what I'm surrounded by, I have to carry a gun.

LISTENER: Considering where you live, you feel you need protection.

OFFENDER: I'm not the one with the problem. If I get high, it's because my family is always nagging me.

LISTENER: You have problems in your family.

communicate the value and worth of the client's view. Keep the focus on the offender client and try not to use patterned prefaces. The minimal prompts of *when, then, you,* or *it* will keep you on the right track.

In sum, keep your reflections simple, and keep yourself out of them. The focus should be on the client. Reflective statements can be quite uncomplicated and straightforward. There are three levels of reflection: repetition, simple, and complex. We'll review the first two here but will save complex reflections for Chapter 6, where they are described within the context of engaging the client.

Repetition

Sometimes the mere repetition of a word or short phrase communicates interest and keeps the conversation going. Repetitions are the most basic reflection because they use clients' own words to repeat a part of what they have said. Some examples of repetition are provided in Table 3.2.

Repetitions may assist for several reasons. First, you may not have understood what the client said. You won't always know what the client is trying to communicate, and sometimes it's difficult to even guess. In these situations, you can remain in the conversation by repeating what the client has said until you can regain traction. Repetitions keep

TABLE 3.2. Repetitions as Reflective Statements

Client statement	Repetition from listener	Simple reflection
"I'm feeling pretty depressed today."	"You're feeling depressed." "It's depressing right now."	"It's bad today; you're feeling low." "You're really down."
"I just don't want to go to that program. It's a waste of my time."	"You don't want to go to that program."	"This is not something that you think will help."
"It's not my fault! My brother is the reason it happened!"	"It's not your fault, but your brother's."	"People are trying to put the blame on you, but that's not where it belongs."
"I feel like I'll never get a job. Who wants to hire someone in my situation?"	"You feel like you'll never get a job with your situation."	"With all that you have going on, you don't think you can be successful."

engagement and rapport building going until we can better understand. Second, you may find your attention drifting during the conversation. This happens to everyone, particularly when it involves a topic you've heard before. When you notice yourself in a moment of inattention, you can use repetition to rejoin the conversation. Third, when dealing with a particularly anxious client, or one with pressured, rapid-fire speech, repetition can slow down the conversation and accentuate points that merit further exploration. This can also help decrease the client's agitation or anxiety, often prompted by their belief that they have to quickly "get it all out" and tell the whole story. Once the client realizes that the listener is attending to him or her, such worry may decrease naturally.

Repetition is the most basic level of reflection. Repetitive statements can be useful, but try not to use them too much, as they may seem mechanical and programmed and will advance the conversation only so far. Other forms of reflection may be helpful as the conversation becomes more complex.

Simple Reflections

With a simple reflection, you repeat or only minimally paraphrase what the client has just said. Refer again to Table 3.2, where each statement contains a repetition as well as a simple reflection. For a moment, picture an iceberg. We can only see a bit of the iceberg at the surface of the water. Likewise, a simple reflection is limited to the content that has been expressed. Another form of reflection—complex reflection—involves the meaning that lies beneath, to be covered further in Chapter 6. But don't overlook the value in simple reflection—this surface view of the problem is important and yet difficult to master.

An important point is to reflect *themes* rather than specific words or phrases. A theme is a key idea or issue embedded in the client's story. Try to find the theme rather than use the client's exact words. For example, the client worried about finding a job in Table 3.2 has noted that it feels like someone in his or her situation will never get a job. Rather than honing in on words like *job* or *situation,* a simple reflection calls for recognizing the theme of "I won't be successful." Other thematic messages may include: "What I try won't matter"; "Everything is stacked against me"; or "I'll never get to where I want to be." Reflecting such themes allows you to accurately paraphrase what the offender has expressed without unnecessary repetition, while also demonstrating that you are engaged and attentive to the meaning of the conversation.

TABLE 3.3. Transforming Questions into Simple Reflections

Question	Simple reflection
"Do you mean that you think nothing's going to help?"	"You feel nothing's going to help." "Nothing will help."
"So you believe that your circumstances will sabotage what you do?"	"Your circumstances will get in the way of what you can do."
"Do you mean that your condition puts employment out of your reach right now?"	"You feel like your condition puts employment out of your reach right now."

Also critical is the urge to ask questions. Asking questions connotes interest. However, a question is not a reflective statement. Instead, you can turn the question into a simple reflection. Returning to our example above, several questions might occur to the listener regarding the offender's fear that he or she will be unable to get a job. Such questions may provide fodder for good reflections, as noted in Table 3.3.

This may seem like a great deal of mental effort for one reflection, and it is. Reflective listening can be hard work at first, and it is more difficult than just asking questions. But like most skills, it becomes easier with practice. Because questioning is less demanding than listening, it is easy to fall into the question–answer trap, asking a series of questions instead of following and reflecting the person's statements. Yet such a pattern may actually evoke defensiveness. Remember, then, that skillful listening is less about extracting information and more about engaging the speaker, keeping the conversation moving forward, and gaining an understanding of the speaker's world.

Learning How to Listen and Reflect

Those who work with offenders vary widely in training and experience. Some have had formal training in counseling and therapy, while others have focused more on procedural or legal matters. Each background is valuable, and the goal here is not to negate what you may have already learned. Instead, one should have a variety of skills, and in using MI, learning to listen deeply is key. Professional listening exists along a continuum, as shown in Figure 3.1. On one end is silent absorbing, where the listener is quiet, yet attentive. Toward the center of the continuum is nonverbal communication, which more actively shows the speaker that

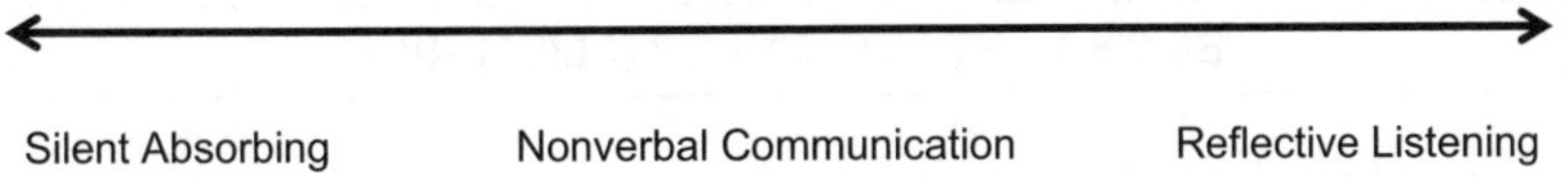

←——————————————————————————————→

Silent Absorbing   Nonverbal Communication   Reflective Listening

FIGURE 3.1. The continuum of professional listening.

he or she has your attention. At the other end we find reflective listening, engaging the speaker in a continuous dialogue.

Each point on this continuum is a skill that can be learned and practiced. To best learn any complex skill, you need feedback—preferably immediate feedback in the moment. Listening thus presents a great opportunity for learning, as it is a dynamic and responsive process. This is especially true of reflections. Each time you offer a reflection, you receive immediate feedback from the speaker about its accuracy and the status of the conversation. Missing the mark is fine—when you're wrong, the speaker will correct you and then tell you more. As you learn, you will have many opportunities to practice, and to see improvements in your guesses at what the speaker means.

The payoff for such practice is vast. If your reflections are accurate, they convey a deep understanding of the speaker's experience. Few offenders have experienced this level of understanding and acceptance. It has a powerful effect, leaving the speaker feeling heard, understood, and wanting to disclose more. To the degree that clients see themselves accurately reflected in your responses, they are likely to fill in the larger picture.

> *Accurate reflections leave the speaker feeling heard, understood, and wanting to disclose more.*

ROADBLOCKS TO LISTENING

Common impressions of listening involve being quiet (at least for a little while) and hearing what the other person has to say. The critical element in reflective or deep listening, however, is what the listener says in response to the speaker. Thus far we have been describing what good listening is. It is equally important, though, to think about what good listening is not. Gordon (1970) identified 12 roadblocks to listening, as listed in Box 3.1.

These roadblocks get in the way of self-exploration and also derail the speaker from his or her natural flow of thought. Further, roadblocks

---

BOX 3.1. ROADBLOCKS TO LISTENING

1. Ordering, directing, or commanding

2. Warning, cautioning, or threatening

3. Giving advice, making suggestions, or providing solutions

4. Persuading with logic, arguing, or lecturing

5. Telling people what they should do; moralizing

6. Disagreeing, judging, criticizing, or blaming

7. Agreeing, approving, or praising

8. Shaming, ridiculing, or labeling

9. Interpreting or analyzing

10. Reassuring, sympathizing, or consoling

11. Questioning or probing

12. Withdrawing, distracting, humoring, or changing the subject

---

imply a power differential in the relationship, with the conversation centered more on the listener than the speaker. The underlying message is "Listen to me. I know best." Consider, for example, a well-intentioned but unhelpful correctional officer talking with an inmate who feels conflicted about quitting his or her use of street drugs. Their conversation, reflected in Box 3.2, also includes designation of specific roadblocks.

From this, one can clearly see that the correctional officer is engaged in the conversation and likely believes his or her responses will help the inmate make a decision about change. Nothing the officer has said is explicitly wrong, but these statements create roadblocks—roadblocks that the inmate must now navigate in order to move forward in the conversation. Importantly, the inmate has not been fully understood, and we have no real understanding of the nature of the person's dilemma. The inmate has been prematurely pushed toward a single resolution without coming to this point on his or her own. The officer hasn't truly listened. In a different situation, any of these statements might have their proper place. But such roadblocks do not represent deep listening, or the level of listening and engagement necessary for MI.

**BOX 3.2. SAMPLE CONVERSATION
WITH ROADBLOCKS TO LISTENING**

OFFENDER: I just don't know whether I can stop using heroin or not.

CORRECTIONAL OFFICER: You should stop. You could get more time behind bars! [#2—warning, cautioning]

OFFENDER: But that's the point! I'm not sure if can stop!

CORRECTIONAL OFFICER: Yes, you can. People quit every day. [#6—disagreeing]

OFFENDER: Well, I just feel trapped . . . like I get locked into using.

CORRECTIONAL OFFICER: Have you thought about treatment, giving yourself a chance? [#3—giving advice, making suggestions]

OFFENDER: Yea, but it's not easy to do treatment, and I'm not sure I want to.

CORRECTIONAL OFFICER: But if you don't do it, you could be wasting your life. [#2—warning, cautioning]

OFFENDER: I don't want to waste away, but it's just not that easy.

CORRECTIONAL OFFICER: It's just what you have to do to take care of yourself. [#4—persuading with logic, lecturing]

OFFENDER: I just don't know how. How will I manage?

CORRECTIONAL OFFICER: You can do it. You'll be fine. You'll see. [#10—reassuring]

MOVING THE CONVERSATION FORWARD

Listening is a foundational element of successful MI. It allows you to develop accurate empathy, to find acceptance, and to build a partnership moving forward. When all else fails, *listen*. But what else? The next step beyond good listening is good interviewing. MI is complex. While the conversation is not about you, you are still a part of it. So in our next chapter, before we move into the core processes of MI, we will talk about interviewing itself. This will set the stage for all else in our conversations about change.

CHAPTER 4

THE ART OF INTERVIEWING

The thing I hate about an argument is that it always interrupts
a discussion.
—G. K. CHESTERTON

MI represents a departure from traditional offender services, but one
that can bring energy and fresh new vision to the field. It speaks to a way
of helping that embodies new values and new practices. After decades of
unique attention to supervision, pressure, and control, MI fosters interest in offender engagement, human motivation, and lifestyle transformation. The opening chapters of this book have covered topics like deep
listening, partnership, compassion, facilitation of strengths, and client
autonomy. These are processes that do not implant ideas into the minds
of offenders but instead evoke thoughts *from* them. Through the spirit
of MI and the practice of skillful listening, offender agencies can return
to the business of behavior change.

In the previous chapter, we explored methods of listening. Now we
move to methods of interviewing. Here, we will talk about some basic
definitions associated with conversations about change, when to use MI,
and important traps that can demotivate both practitioners and clients.

THE ART OF INTERVIEWING:
CONVERSATIONS ABOUT CHANGE

Modus operandi is a Latin phrase that means "method of operation."
Often heard in the context of criminal profiling or investigation, it connotes that offenders may have habits or patterns of behavior that help

identify them across situations. Interestingly, there is also a modus operandi that characterizes work with offenders. Whether it is case management, supervision, therapy, risk assessment, or other evaluative decision making, the common thread across these many contexts is conversation. *We talk*—a steady stream of dialogue emerges with the shared goal of finding answers that will prevent future unlawful behavior. And when talking fails, we're left with expensive alternatives like court hearings, increased levels of supervision, and even incarceration.

These expensive practices drain our patience, energy, and agency resources. They mean doing more of what has already been largely unsuccessful in promoting change. However, as an alternative approach, MI can turn argumentative and defensive encounters with offenders into conversations about change. While not a cure-all, MI is a helpful method to assist offenders with identifying their own reasons for change. It offers real choice, all in the context of our usual modus operandi—conversation.

This is juxtaposed with genuine frustration on the part of staff, officers, and therapists who work with offenders and find that many simply parrot the right words and do "just enough" to get people to leave them alone. This is certainly not true behavior change. MI provides the opportunity to work toward something beyond acquiescence. An old joke from musicians seems apt: "It doesn't cost us any more to play in tune." For us, it doesn't cost any more to talk about behavior change.

> *MI can turn argumentative and defensive encounters with offenders into conversations about change.*

A THOUGHTFUL EXPERIMENT

Try this thought experiment, or better still, try it with a friend or colleague. Choose something that you could, should, want to, or need to change, but haven't yet. It could be a health-related or other lifestyle change, a negative habit, an opportunity for something new, or something involving your work. Now imagine (or have) a "helper" who tells you: (1) how much you need to make this change, (2) all of the reasons for doing so, (3) why it's so important to change, (4) how to do it, (5) how likely it is that you can do it, and (6) how easy it is to just set your mind to it and make it happen.

How would you likely respond? In offender agency trainings across the globe, people's responses are remarkably consistent. A small few find it helpful—perhaps 1 in 20, which may be just enough to keep it in practice—but most often the person "helped" feels some, if not all, of the following:

- Angry (agitated, annoyed, irritated, not heard, not understood)
- Defensive (discounting, judged, justifying, oppositional, unwilling to change)
- Uncomfortable (ashamed, overwhelmed, eager to leave)
- Powerless (passive, one-down, discouraged, disengaged)

In fact, sometimes the person being "helped" concludes that he or she *doesn't* want to make the change after all! That was never the intention, of course. It's merely how people normally respond to being told what, how, and why they should change. In response to these directives, people most often feel bad. And feeling bad doesn't inspire change.

Imagine further how the interview would have gone if the "helper" had used muscle—the authoritarian "I'm in control" demeanor so common to offender-based work. When you meet, the person helping you refuses to shake your hand. He or she peppers you with questions that force a yes or no answer, and you find yourself unable to express your opinion or explain your side of the story. During the conversation, you're told, "You better do this," or "I'm in charge here, not you!" The "helper" rolls his or her eyes in frustration when you offer your ideas, and then looks to the ceiling in obvious disgust when you say that you're not sure you're ready to change. It worsens when you say you don't know if you want to change at all. Imagine your reaction as the speaker. It's likely not positive, or in favor of change. The number of persons who might have found the original conversation helpful drops dramatically, while anger, combativeness, and unwillingness increase.

Now try it again, but this time a bit differently. Again, imagine something that you could, should, want to, or need to change but haven't yet. This time, your friend or colleague gives you no advice at all but instead asks you a series of questions, listening respectfully to what you say. These are four questions developed by Miller and Rollnick (2013) to give beginners a feeling for MI.

1. "Why would you want to make this change?"
2. "How might you go about it in order to succeed?"

3. "What are the three best reasons for you to do it?"
4. "How important is it for you to make this change, and why?"

After listening patiently, the "helper" gives a short summary of what *you* have said, including why you want to change, why it's important, what the best reasons are, and how you could do it in order to succeed. Then there is one final question:

5. "So what do you think you'll do?"

That's all. We haven't yet explained what's going on in this conversation about change, or given you any guidelines. Nor, however, have we made assumptions. The questions themselves are not the method, but they do provide a sense of the person-centered style of MI. In contrast to the first imagined or practiced conversation, people who have experienced this latter method typically feel otherwise afterward:

- Engaged (interested, cooperative, liking the listener, ready to keep talking)
- Empowered (able to change, hopeful, optimistic)
- Open (accepted, comfortable, safe, respected)
- Understood (connected, heard, listened to)

In both instances the subject of the conversation is the same—a possible change characterized by ambivalence—but the outcomes are quite different. So who would you rather work with? Angry, defensive, uncomfortable, and passive people who don't like you, or people who feel engaged, empowered, open, and understood, and who rather like the time they spent with you? They are the *same people*. The difference is in the conversation.

A DEFINITION OF MI

This is a process called "motivational interviewing." The word *motivational* seems straightforward enough. It's about motivation. But what about *interviewing*? The word *interview* is different from words like *therapy* or *counseling*. An interview suggests fairness—an opportunity to be heard. There are fewer assumptions about power or roles specific to the interaction. An interview conveys a partnership of sorts: an employer interviews a new hire, with both roles critical in filling a vacant position. In some contexts, the interviewer or listener is in the one-down position, with something to gain from the speaker. Beat reporters might interview famous or newsworthy people. Students interview experts to enhance their education. The reporter and the student are both interested audiences, eager to learn. Important here is that both are working together (thus, "inter-"), viewing things from a shared perspective.

With the foundation in place, we begin to define MI. Let us offer three definitions of increasing complexity. *First, it is a way to help people find their own reasons for change.* This definition is one that resonates with clients and laypersons who merely want to know what MI is. *Second, it is a way to strategically use questions and statements to help people think and talk in a positive direction* (Miller & Rollnick, 2013). This subsequent definition begins to explain how we might use MI: it is a process of getting people to talk about change. *Finally, MI is a person-centered, goal-oriented method of communication that elicits and strengthens intrinsic motivation for positive change* (Miller & Rollnick, 2013). Now we have the "why" of MI. We use it because it strengthens the person's own motivation for change, and it places us in the role of one who facilitates change.

WHEN GOALS DIFFER—THE TIME FOR MI

By now, you may have a better idea of what MI is, as well as what it isn't. You know why you might want to use it. But still, a common question from those learning MI, particularly with offenders, is *when* to use it. We've talked about a new mind-set and heart-set, or the idea that we should approach offenders in a different spirit (Chapter 2). However, that's not the answer to this question. We also know that listening and reflecting (Chapter 3) are critical components of the process, though that doesn't answer the question either. The real answer to this question begins here. As you listen, and as you move further into the conversation about change, you will discover the person's goals. The offender has goals. It is also quite likely that you, or your agency, have goals. In Figure 4.1, we provide a simple grid to illustrate what happens when our goals differ.

For situations involving Cells A and D, there is no apparent problem. Your goals and the offender's goals align. Most counselors who see voluntary clients can expect what we see in Cell A. For example, a client may enter a therapist's office and say, "I want to work on my marriage."

		Is this the current goal of the offender?	
		Yes	No
Is this your current goal for the offender?	Yes	A	B
	No	C	D

Cell A: You and the offender agree on the current goal.

Cell B: You have a goal for the offender that he or she does not share.

Cell C: The offender's goal is not one that you want to prioritize or address at this time.

Cell D: You and the offender agree that the target or topic is not a current goal.

FIGURE 4.1. Possible combinations of our and offenders' goals.

Agreement is realized in the first meeting. Probation officers may occasionally experience this when the offender completely capitulates: "I want to get off probation, and *if you to tell me what to do, I'll do it!*" If this is really how the probationer feels and exactly what he or she wants, behavior change may begin without much discussion or exploration. MI may still play a role, particularly given that even persons in Cell A may experience ambivalence, setbacks, or lack of support. In Cell D, you and the offender agree that a specific goal is unnecessary, or that perhaps it is a lesser priority than other, more important goals. Perhaps it is a goal that has already been achieved. Or it is a goal that, while interesting, lacks an element of immediacy. This, too, is a situation that does not call for the use of MI.

In Cell C, the offender has a goal that you do not share. Maybe this is a goal that falls outside of your area of expertise, the scope of offender supervision and management, or what you are able to provide in the way of treatment. Such a discrepancy or difference in goals could reflect your ethical discomfort with the offender's goal, or inability to commit to the offender's goal for some other reason. You may not have another goal in mind. In such situations, you may make an appropriate referral, or collaborate with others who are more able to address those aspects of the offender's needs.

This leaves Cell B, a scenario in which you have identified a goal that the offender does not yet share. This is common when clients are required to participate in treatment by the courts or other agencies, including probation, voluntary admission to a facility as a diversionary measure, or also when clients are seeking help for other reasons but not explicitly because of the root problem (e.g., emergency-room care for an alcohol-related injury). These are the situations for which

MI was originally developed—when the offender is *ambivalent* about change, and beyond ambivalence may also harbor a sense of uncertainty and even defensiveness. Ambivalence, a concept discussed further in Chapters 7 and 8, occurs when the offender's beliefs simultaneously support and counter the need for change. There are two or more sides to the argument, which may be felt by the offender as a tug-of-war. With MI, you highlight the offender's own motivations and facilitate decision making about change.

> *With MI, you highlight the offender's own motivations and facilitate decision making about change.*

However, also in Cell B are those who have no ambivalence about change. Some offenders simply do not want to change, or they see no need for it. Prochaska, DiClemente, and Norcross (1992b) hypothesized stages of change, in which this lack of ambivalence is characterized as precontemplation. The offender has yet to consider the downside to his or her problem behavior, though you see a reason to work toward change. So what do you do?

One approach in addictions treatment has been to say, "Come back when you're ready to make changes." This is not the only choice available to substance abuse counselors—you need not wait for clients to "hit rock bottom" or find their motivation before intervening in a helpful way (Meyers & Wolfe, 2004; Miller, Meyers, & Tonigan, 1999; Sellman, Sullivan, Dore, Adamson, & MacEwan, 2001). It may, however, be easier for the helping professional to see only self-motivated clients. In offender work, a parallel concept is identifying offender clients as either friends or enemies. This presents as a dichotomous rule for new offender clients: "If you follow the rules, we'll be friends and get along fine. But if you don't, we'll proceed as enemies." The implicit (or maybe explicit) message for the offender is that all change is up to him or her, and that staff members, therapists, or case managers are merely passive observers of the process. To us, it represents a fatalistic view of change—change agents are helplessly dependent on forces beyond their control. In addition, it is a view that emphasizes compliance. Neither view positions you to influence positive change.

Another approach for offenders and offender service personnel who find themselves in Cell B is to apply pressure, or to exert authoritarian influence to force the offender into agreement on a shared goal. Perhaps in part due to the desire to perform well in their jobs and see good outcomes for their clients, and also in part due to frustration, many offender service providers pressure offenders into accepting a change goal because they "know what's best." While it is true that objective observers may be able to see alternatives or possibilities that the offender doesn't, it is also true that the person knows his or her own needs and capabilities better than anyone else (as we have described in Chapter 2). Exercising pressure to resolve the discrepancy between your goal and the offender's goal is unlikely to result in successful behavior change. Instead, MI can help align the offender's and service provider's goals.

The process of MI is helpful when goals differ but also when ambivalence is blocking the way for the offender to be successful. Importantly, MI is not simply the means through which to make the offender acquiesce to your goals. It is a way of having a conversation about change that clarifies goals and expectations, and that creates a shared perspective between you and the offender client.

ADVANCING THE INTERVIEW

In the previous chapter, we examined professional listening. The continuum of listening described within Chapter 3 ranged from silent absorption of information on one end to active, reflective listening on the other. In this chapter, we examine interviewing as a reciprocal exchange of information. Respectful and thoughtful back-and-forth communication champions the offender's autonomy and needs. The alternative—a one-way flow of information—calls for you to simply tell the offender what to do. Such an approach often leads to a disengaged, frustrated, and unmotivated client. Instead, we want an interviewing style that advances the conversation, keeps the offender engaged and motivated, and results in more positive behavior change.

To illustrate this, we offer two brief exchanges in contrasting interview styles. In these examples, a man under the supervision of the probation office has been detained by the local police following a violent altercation with his wife. He was not arrested but instead escorted away from his home for the evening, and the responding officers contacted his probation officer. In Boxes 4.1 and 4.2 are two possible conversations that might occur during a meeting between this man and his probation officer. Interview 1 (see Box 4.1) includes common interviewing pitfalls that may be familiar to the reader well versed in traditional offender practices. In interview 2 (see Box 4.2), we see an exchange that is more clearly consistent with the spirit and practice of MI.

Take a look at each of these interviews. In the first, the offender client

---

BOX 4.1. INTERVIEW 1:
TRADITIONAL OFFENDER INTERVIEWING STYLE

OFFENDER: I'm going to tell you right now that it's my *wife* who should be sitting here today, not me.

PROBATION OFFICER: It sounds like you fight quite a bit. How often do you two argue like that?

OFFENDER: Well, I'm not the cause of it, if that's what you mean. She needs to share the blame, but the police never see it that way.

PROBATION OFFICER: The responding officer said he didn't think you were in control of your anger. How often does that happen to you?

OFFENDER: Well I don't know . . . sometimes before payday. She gets on my nerves about our bills.

PROBATION OFFICER: And how about other times during the week?

OFFENDER: Well, sometimes in the evening when we're both tired. Probably a couple times a week.

PROBATION OFFICER: So several times a week. And how bad does your fighting get?

OFFENDER: Usually just yelling. Sometimes I break things or punch the walls.

PROBATION OFFICER: That sounds like it gets physical, too. Do you also argue like this when your children are home?

OFFENDER: Sometimes, yeah. But a lot of times they're in bed. They're asleep, so they don't know.

PROBATION OFFICER: I see. A lot of times children say they hear their parents fighting after they've gone to bed. They would hear things, and they'd be scared.

OFFENDER: Well, I don't always punch the walls or throw things. You just don't understand how my wife can get. She won't stop until she's got me going crazy.

PROBATION OFFICER: And do you leave the room, or try to get away from her, do anything to deescalate the situation?

OFFENDER: Wait, why does this always have to be on me? I'm telling you she's part of the problem!

PROBATION OFFICER: But your anger outbursts . . . you've said before that they've been a problem in your marriage for over 2 years.

OFFENDER: I don't know. Maybe. Did I say 2 years? Might not have been that long. And it's not usually this much of a problem. She overreacted and called the police this time.

PROBATION OFFICER: Do you think that you have a problem with anger?

OFFENDER: No, not really. If my wife would back off, none of this would happen.

> PROBATION OFFICER: Well, I need to tell you something. Your display of physical violence is way beyond what's appropriate, and far more than the vast majority of husbands and fathers. Your inability to back off and break off when things get tense tells me your anger gets the best of you. You're putting your wife and your children in danger, and I think you need to take another anger management group to learn more about destressing your life. This one should be the "extended" group because this is just going to keep on getting worse.
>
> OFFENDER: Well, I don't agree. Here we go again. I knew you wouldn't really understand.

is defensive, less open to the conversation, and ends with little motivation to continue the conversation, or to change. In fact, he states several times that he does not need to change. In the second, the client keeps talking, relates information he has learned in his treatment group, and ends with a desire for more. What's different? They both begin in the same manner, and the client is the same person. In the first, the interviewing probation officer asks closed questions, makes judgments about the client, and ends with an authoritarian pronouncement. In the second, however, the officer listens, reflects, and uses a reciprocal, guiding style of communication that will be explored more fully in Chapters 5 and 6. Consider further the contrast between the two interviews in relation to these questions:

- Who voices the argument for change?
- What do you think the probation officer is thinking or feeling?
- What do you think the offender client is thinking or feeling?
- Is engagement enhanced or diminished?
- Is there a common goal in this interview?
- How likely is the offender to change after this interview?

As you contemplate these, keep in mind that there are ways of advancing the interview, just as there are ways of becoming trapped. Both are important. We now turn to a discussion of potential pitfalls or traps in interviewing that can disrupt the flow of the conversation and subvert motivation for change.

INTERVIEWING TRAPS

Working with offenders can be a difficult job. We face multiple demands, complex responsibilities, and conflicting goals and priorities. Our job is

---

BOX 4.2. INTERVIEW 2: AN MI STYLE

OFFENDER: I'm going to tell you right now that it's my *wife* who should be sitting here today, not me.

PROBATION OFFICER: You feel she has a lot to do with this.

OFFENDER: Well, the police don't see it that way.

PROBATION OFFICER: The police seem to take her side.

OFFENDER: Yeah, she pushes and pushes. Nags at me about bills . . . and about the kids. I work hard, and she doesn't see that.

PROBATION OFFICER: It sounds like you try hard to be a good provider, even in a tough situation.

OFFENDER: Yeah, you know? But a lot of the time she doesn't stop until I've gone ballistic! I just don't know where this is all going to end. I feel so stressed, like there's no end to it.

PROBATION OFFICER: If we take a step back from it all for a moment, tell me what you know about stress and how it affects people.

OFFENDER: Well, I learned in my class that stress is like water in a glass, and if your glass is always full to the top, even a little drop of water added to it will make it all spill over.

PROBATION OFFICER: You've got a good understanding of why someone's anger can spill over.

OFFENDER: Right. I mean, I know that I'm walking around with my glass too full. There's just so much, all of the time.

PROBATION OFFICER: Your wife, or any situation that causes stress, really . . . and your glass is full already. So you explode. You don't like that.

OFFENDER: Exactly. Who wants to be walking around ready to snap? I don't like it.

PROBATION OFFICER: I wonder if I might tell you some things that I've noticed with other people who were struggling with too much stress?

OFFENDER: All right.

PROBATION OFFICER: When people know their glass is too full, they have to find ways to pour water out of the glass. Some people take walks, some try to work out, or if they're too tired after a day of work, they find some quiet time. If life gets too busy to allow that, then they arrange something with their partner like a time-out in an argument. It gives them a break to move to different rooms, leave the house for few minutes, walk around, or do anything to break off for a few minutes. How does that sound to you?

OFFENDER: My class mentioned some of these. We made fun of some of them, but you're saying that I should start using some of these ideas?

PROBATION OFFICER: You could. I know it sounds hard because you're already so busy, but it's like getting enough antibiotic medication in you when

> you're sick. When you have enough of a dose in you, you immediately start feeling a little better. Only with stress, it's emptying it out of you. Dumping some water out of your glass before your wife and what's at home pours more in.
>
> OFFENDER: I've got to find a way to deal with this stress. I didn't think I needed the class. I thought I could do it myself.
>
> PROBATION OFFICER: You realize that the stress is stronger than you thought.
>
> OFFENDER: In class, they had this saying: "Stress seldom takes vacations." Boy, they had that right. I work my butt off for my family, and this happens? It's not what I want. How do I start?

also made difficult by the day-to-day experiences, like the heartache, the hurt, fractured families, disheveled lives, despair, hopelessness, violence, and suffering. We appreciate and admire those who choose this work. A life of service to others is a profound gift. People may choose this work for any number of selfless motives—a desire to give back, to prevent and alleviate suffering, to manifest spirituality or love of their fellow human beings, or to make a positive difference in the lives of others and in the world.

Ironically, these same motives can lead to problems when the task is to help people change. Helpers want to help, and when something or someone is out of balance, there is a powerful urge to restore that balance. Seeing people head down the wrong path, there is a natural desire to get in front of them and say, "Stop! Go back! Don't you see? Your path will lead to ruin! There is a better way!" It is done with the best of intentions. This is called the "righting reflex," or the desire to fix what appears wrong and promptly set the person on a better course. And many view offenders, as a group, as those who may need more "righting" than others. The righting reflex however does more than push us to fix the problem. It also drives our approach to the interview. When you perceive that the offender isn't listening to your advice, you confront the client with reality, provide the obvious solution, and turn up the volume, making your points in a repetitive, directive, and authoritarian manner (White & Miller, 2007).

The righting reflex is a profound barrier to effective interviewing. Trying to set people aright has the paradoxical effect of only making them more firmly entrenched in their original position. And in response, there is the temptation to simply apply more pressure. This runs counter to the goal of change and is inconsistent with an MI style. The righting reflex, though, is not the only interviewing trap that moves us further from a conversation about change. Other messages, particularly those that assert one's authority or promote client passivity, also threaten client engagement. Let us consider six such traps.

The Assessment Trap

This problematic style can emerge even during the first interview session. In many offender agencies or facilities, the intake session involves a structured assessment format. The staff person asks questions, and the offender answers them. The offender is immediately relegated to a passive role, asked to defend his or her decisions and recount a story that is often already known to the interviewer. The speaker has little power and is alienated from the start. The offender may believe that all sessions will proceed in the same manner and quickly disengage.

Why does this happen? First, there is pressure to gather information. The reality, though, is that usually you already have what you need, and the offender will provide the rest if you take time to listen to the story rather than directing it yourself. Second, you mistakenly think that if you ask enough questions, you'll know what to do. This is rarely true, and it is not solely up to you to figure out what to do. Finally, this pattern of questions and answers sometimes results from anxiety, whether yours or the offender's. Indeed, staff anxiety is associated with less empathic responding and prompts a structured question–answer format (Rubino, Barker, Roth, & Fearon, 2000). The staff person controls the session by asking questions, while the client is forced to respond with short, direct answers. Here is a brief example:

> INTERVIEWER: You're here because of domestic violence issues—is that right?
>
> CLIENT: Yes.
>
> INTERVIEWER: Do you think you have a hard time controlling your anger?
>
> CLIENT: Probably.
>
> INTERVIEWER: What sets you off? Your wife?
>
> CLIENT: Mostly, yeah.
>
> INTERVIEWER: Have you ever gone overboard when arguing?
>
> CLIENT: Lately, yes.

It happens so easily, yet this creates problems. For one, it teaches the person to give short, simple answers rather than the elaboration needed for MI and behavior change. Also, it sets an expectation of expert helper versus passive offender. There is little opportunity for people to direct the conversation to explore their own motivation or voice reasons for change. The offender's role in the relationship is limited to answering questions. In such an exchange, the client has little chance of genuine expression. It also sets the stage for the next obstacle—the expert trap.

The Expert Trap

In some situations, a client may seek or expect expert advice. We want expert advice from a ski instructor during a first skiing lesson. When we pay expensive rates for an attorney's expertise, we're not usually looking for a "shared voice" in his or her answers—we pay for the attorney's legal opinion. Certainly this is also the case when we see a physician for an acute need. We expect to leave with a diagnosis or informed medical opinion, as well as perhaps a prescription or advice on how to treat the ailment. In each of these examples, there is an established presumption of expertise and an accepted power differential in the relationship.

With regard to personal change, the expert role works less well. A prescription of "just do this" is seldom effective, and the provider's consequent frustration is "I tell them, and I tell them, *and I tell them,* and still they don't change!" Part of MI is recognizing that you will only find the right path for each offender client through collaboration and acknowledgment of the client's expertise. You are an expert in many ways. You have professional training, knowledge, and years of experience. Still, the client knows him- or herself better than you do, despite these things. It's a freeing experience. *You don't have to know everything.* Your job is to let the offender do the talking and tell you what works best for him or her.

Helping professionals should take a "not-knowing" posture with clients (Anderson & Goolishian, 1992). Such an approach means that while we do have areas of knowledge relevant to offender change— the effects of criminality and drug use, what constitutes increased risk, available treatment options or community resources, or systemic responses to continued problem behavior—we can set these aside during the conversation to become patient and interested listeners. Only the offender can know the intricacies of his or her own life and current situation, hopes for a better future, or priorities and needs. Further, the offender is the only one who really knows when he or she has changed, or what it may take to get there. By suspending our knowledge, as well as our desire to express that knowledge, we will learn and accomplish more.

The Premature Focus Trap

It is quite tempting to identify and hone in on the offender's "real" prob-lem. This isn't necessarily the problem that the person wanted to talk about, but instead what you or someone else (e.g., the court, others in your agency) has determined is the foremost priority for change. Herein lies a critical problem: Until offenders have decided that change is impor-tant (the "why"), they are uninterested in the steps they must take to get there (the "how"). The helper often assumes that the offender will see why change is necessary, leaving behind the need to ensure that the offender is in agreement. It's like an old vaudeville routine where two people tied together back to back try to head in opposite directions.

This trap is a variation of the righting reflex. You offer informa-tion about potentially dire consequences of behavior in order to shock a client into awareness or compliance. While such information may be correct, it may not be helpful. For example, imagine saying, "Your blood-alcohol content was beyond 'super drunk.' You could have died!" This statement makes the mistake of telling the client what he or she should be concerned about, rather than evoking the client's own con-cerns. What's more, it leads to persistent effort to draw the person back to the "real" problem without listening to the offender's other concerns. A struggle ensues, and it is unlikely that the offender will change. The point is to avoid becoming too committed to a goal or topic early in the interview. Start with the client's concerns. Listen to the story. Gain a broader understanding of the client's life, and at some point you may be able to return to the topic you need to discuss, having acquired a great deal more along the way.

The Labeling Trap

Based upon the assessment and premature focus traps, when you iden-tify and want to focus on a particular problem, you are also tempted to name it. Assessments produce a diagnosis. One assumes that the diag-nosis should be the focus of treatment. Some believe that it is terribly important for a person to accept or even admit the diagnosis and may resort to rather accusatory labels: "You have anger issues"; "You're an alcoholic"; "You're in denial"; "You've been diagnosed with depres-sion." Because such labels often carry stigma and elicit shame, it is not surprising that people resist them.

A complex interpersonal dynamic underlies the labeling trap. The listener, rather than just listening, is attempting to assert control and expertise. Labels serve as evidence to turn the offender to your way of thinking. The speaker, however, may perceive this as judgment and condemnation. Even a seemingly harmless reference to "your problem with . . . " can elicit uncomfortable feelings of being criticized. The danger, of course, is that such labeling evokes discord and so-called lines being drawn. Progress and change don't have "sides," and with the imposition of labels, sides are established, and progress is hindered.

In contrast, problems can be fully explored without attaching labels to them. In some cases, the client enters with a label that he or she embraces and identifies with. If it is helpful to the person, there is little need to wrest it away. However, you also need not embrace the label fully yourself, as doing so may prevent you from seeing and evoking the person's entire sense of being. It is easy to miss problems when you too easily focus on just one. Often, however, the offender client may raise the issue of having been previously assessed and labeled in a way that suggests he or she is unhappy with it. How you respond is quite important. We recommend a combination of reflecting and reframing—concepts that will be explored throughout this text. This is illustrated in a brief example in Box 4.3.

Consider, too, that labels are insidious and may change people's behavior, as well as our way of viewing them. Call someone a psychopath, antisocial, or deviant, and he or she becomes so. Our own private labels for offenders, sometimes shared with colleagues—*pervert, loser, creep*—can be even more derogatory than what the official assessment provides, and such terms create distance between you and the person you're working with. Labels establish pessimistic expectations, causing you to doubt people, their environment, and their ability to cope with the issues at hand. The humanistic spirit of MI, as examined in Chapter 2, can counteract the damage caused by labeling.

The Blaming Trap

As early as the first session, the client may become mired in defensiveness and blaming. *Whose fault is it? Who's to blame for this?* It is easy to fall into this way of thinking. It distracts us, though, from our goals. We waste a great deal of time and energy on seeking answers to who is at fault, countering client defensiveness, and even becoming defensive ourselves. One obvious approach is to render blame irrelevant. The court determines guilt or innocence; it is not your responsibility. Once a determination has been made, need you reinforce it in your daily work? Further, you perform assessments and assign labels—both of which can lead to confusion about blame. A person who is "dangerous" sounds clearly guilty. Similarly, a diagnosis of problematic substance use implies difficulty in controlling behavior. This manner of thinking hinders our

---

BOX 4.3. AVOIDING THE LABELING TRAP

CLIENT: So that assessment said I had a problem? Oh, so you think I'm an addict!

INTERVIEWER: It's noted in your substance abuse assessment that's in your legal file, but here in my office, I'm much more concerned about what you think.

CLIENT: Well, I don't like being called an addict. You can use heroin and not be an addict.

INTERVIEWER: When someone calls you that, you want them to know that your situation really isn't that bad.

CLIENT: Well, yes. But I'm not saying that I don't have problems.

INTERVIEWER: But you don't like being called a "problem." It sounds harsh to you.

CLIENT: Yes, it does.

INTERVIEWER: That's pretty common, as you might imagine. I talk to lots of people who don't like being labeled. There's nothing strange about that. I don't like people labeling me, either.

CLIENT: I feel like I'm being put in a box.

INTERVIEWER: Right. So let me tell you how I see this, and then we'll move on. To me, it doesn't matter what we call a problem. We don't have to call it anything. If a label is an important issue for you, we can discuss it, but it's not particularly important to me. What really matters is to understand how your use of heroin is harming you, and what, if anything, you want to do about it. That's what I care about—you.

---

work toward behavior change. Therefore, let us be wary of confusing an assessment with a statement of responsibility.

Blame can emerge from all sides. Offenders may initiate self-blame, which you can address through reflection and reframing. For example:

> "It sounds like sometimes you feel like it's your fault. But you also see that others had a lot to do with what happened. My job, though, isn't to decide who's at fault. That's what a judge does, but not me. I'm not figuring out who's to blame. I'm more concerned with where you are, where you might want to be, and what we can do to get you there."

Primarily, you want to make clear that your role is to help rather than assign blame. Offering a statement to that effect at the beginning may facilitate conversations of growth. Periodic reminders at times when you or the offender experience the urge to address fault or responsibility may help as well.

The Chat Trap

Finally, it is possible to fall into the trap of just chatting with the offender, with little direction to guide the conversation. Making "small talk" can be a friendly way to initiate conversation, and there are benefits to non-intrusive and impersonal conversation to soothe anxious nerves during a first meeting. And indeed, offenders from some cultures consider this a necessity before moving to more serious conversation. Although such chatting may feel comfortable, the benefits fade quickly beyond modest doses. Higher levels of informal chatting in session are predictive of lower levels of client motivation for change, as well as difficulties with retaining changes already made (Bamatter et al., 2010). Similarly, higher frequency of informal discussion is related to less proficiency in MI and poorer in-session change in client motivation (Martino, Ball, Nich, Frankforter, & Carroll, 2009).

The chat trap, therefore, requires a careful balance. Some amount of chatting may be necessary to acknowledge cultural social conventions, and to ease client nerves. It may also decrease your own anxiety during a first meeting. Yet too much chatting is counterproductive for facilitating a conversation about change. Fortunately, training in MI has been associated with significantly less informal discussion in session (Martino et al., 2009). This is perhaps because MI calls us to be mindful and specific in our choices during every conversation. Return to the spirit of MI—if done correctly, the conversation will guide you toward deeper understanding and accurate empathy, both of which are only achieved through genuine rather than superficial interactions with clients.

MOVING FROM CONCEPT TO PRACTICE

In the preceding chapters, we have described the integral components of the spirit of MI, or what keeps us in the proper mind-set and heart-set to do this important work. We have delved into the arts of listening and interviewing, which are so vital to our work with offenders and persons who struggle with their motivation to change. Now we move forward into the *practice* of MI, or the ways in which we implement MI in our moment-by-moment interactions with our offender clients. We begin with engaging, the necessary foundation upon which we can build a collaborative partnership with our clients and work toward behavior change.

CHAPTER 5

ENGAGING

The Relational Foundation

We are afraid to care too much for fear that the other person
does not care at all.
—ELEANOR ROOSEVELT

MI involves four basic processes: engaging, focusing, evoking, and
planning. We begin with engagement, a step that calls us to engage
the offender in a collaborative working relationship. MI places great
emphasis on establishing such a relationship. Treatment research is both
numerous and resolute on this subject; good relationships lead to good
outcomes. Of the many factors that contribute to treatment outcome,
one of the largest is the therapeutic alliance (e.g., Duncan, Best, &
Hagen, 2010; Norcross, 2002). Spanning multiple disciplines and areas
of clinical need, over 1,000 empirical studies have found evidence that
the therapeutic alliance facilitates positive change outcomes (Orlinsky,
Ronnestad, & Willutzki, 2004). Characteristics of these strong alliances
include trust, being aligned with goals, respect for autonomy, and clear
communication of wants and needs (Norcross, 2002).

This alliance is not limited to therapists. The quality of the relationship is also important in teaching, parenting, friendship, health care,
ministry, sales, and many other interactions that can influence change.
Should nontherapists still strive for what has been called a *therapeutic*
alliance? Yes. A strong and beneficial alliance will serve offender clients well, regardless of whether or not you are a therapist. What would
this alliance look like? Working relationship, therapeutic alliance,

collaboration, helping partnership, and simply "alliance" are all used interchangeably. In MI, it is *engagement*. How do you define or measure engagement from the perspective of behavior change? And how might this differ from traditional ideas of how we should relate to offenders? This is certainly a valid question, as outcomes in corrections and other offender service systems have suffered from a historically limited view of the relationship between staff and offender (Clark, 2009). In this tradition, engagement has been reduced to a firm and straightforward explanation of rules, successful only when the offender complies. Behavior change, however welcomed, has long taken a backseat to obedience (Clark, 2005). However, MI redefines our limited view of engagement and expands it to include much more.

Bordin (1979) and Duncan et al. (2003) describe the alliance as an interacting system established between you and the offender that includes three conditions:

1. The development of a relationship bond between you and your client.
2. Agreement on the goals of your work together.
3. Working together on mutually negotiated tasks to reach these goals.

The process of engaging emphasizes the first component of the alliance: the process of establishing a mutually trusting and respectful helping relationship. The latter two components certainly continue to build a positive relationship with the offender, though these are addressed more thoroughly within the context of focusing and evoking (see Chapters 7–10).

From the perspective of the offender, engagement is found in answers to the following questions: "Do I feel respected?"; "Does he or she listen to me and try to understand my ideas?"; "Do I trust this person?"; "Does he or she allow me to have a say in how I comply with court orders, or fulfill my treatment plan?"; "Am I offered options, or is it always a 'one-size-fits-all' approach?"; "Does he or she negotiate with me, rather than dictate the rules?" The answers to these questions are critical, as what is often missing from offender research is the offender's perspective (Farrall, 2002). This is especially troublesome when research has found that the *offender's* evaluation of the alliance—not ours—has proven to be the more accurate predictor of outcomes (Bachelor & Horvath, 1999). Engagement, perhaps, is in the eye of the beholder.

Fostering engagement is not coddling or fluff. It is a meaningful part of moving toward behavior change. It is also more than a series of tools or strategies for ensuring that the offender likes you. That is not the purpose of engagement. Instead, it is the basis upon which any change will occur, and it is expected that you will attend to engagement throughout the process of MI or working with offenders to facilitate rehabilitation and reentry (see Figure 5.1).

The key to building such a foundation of engagement rests in communication with the client. Communication involves more than just talking. It requires a spirit or attitude conducive to acceptance and change. It requires attentive listening. And it requires you to focus on how you frame the things you say. In the following sections, we will discuss important components of engaging the offender, including styles of communication, communication pitfalls, and developing a client-centered approach.

THE THREE STYLES OF COMMUNICATION: DIRECTING, GUIDING, AND FOLLOWING

The styles of conversation with offenders occur along a continuum. At one end is a directing style, characterized by giving advice, setting directions, or providing information. For the most part, those working with offenders are expected to be active and directive toward them. This expectation comes from multiple sources, whether it is the court, a specific offender agency or facility, or the community as a whole. Likewise, the offender is expected to follow and comply with what he or she is directed to do. With a directing style, it is your responsibility to explain the court's orders or communicate the rules, and it is the offender's responsibility to accept your direction. Examples of common directing efforts include serving probation orders, explaining drug-screening urinalysis programs, setting up appointments, or redirecting poor behavior. This is perhaps the style most familiar to those in offender agencies. We fall into it almost by default.

At the other end of the continuum is a following style. This yielding style has its place in offender work as well. Listening and getting to know the clients, placing value on their views, and trying to understand their values and beliefs are indicative of following. You allow the client to lead, taking your cues from his or her conversation. Following certainly has its place, as there are some situations where you have no clear path, or when being directive would be inappropriate or ineffective. For example, an offender may break into tears during an interview

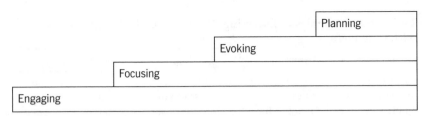

FIGURE 5.1. Engaging as the foundation for the four processes of motivational interviewing. From Miller and Rollnick (2013). Copyright © 2013 The Guilford Press. Reprinted by permission.

for reasons unknown to you, or as the result of strong emotions you do not yet understand. Being directive or giving orders at that moment would seem harsh and inappropriate. It may also elicit a highly negative reaction from the person, hindering future work. The person may feel misunderstood or worse yet, attacked. Instead, you want to listen and solicit further information to find out what prompted the strong emotion, accepting where it takes you. Examples of common following efforts include intake interviews, setting up individualized plans, or discussion of trauma or other sensitive topics. While this style is not always immediately associated with offender work, there are times when following the offender's lead in the conversation is warranted.

Neither directing nor following captures the guiding style that lies between. What does this guiding style look like? Take, for example, teaching a child to ride a bike. Directing involves simply yet abstractly telling him or her the mechanics of foot movement, steering, and balance. Following might resemble watching the child try (and fall) and providing encouragement or waiting to see if the child learns it on his or her own. Guiding, on the other hand, is more complex though infinitely more helpful. Giving suggestions, rather than orders, is more appropriate and sensible. You help new bike riders find wobbly success, or support them when they fall. A skillful guide offers expertise and tips when needed, attentively listens to determine problem areas or needed solutions, and radiates a "can do" attitude, all to help the child succeed. It's this midpoint on the continuum—this guiding style—that best describes MI. A guiding style is most effective for motivating change. All change is self-change, and communicating through guidance best assists skill acquisition and behavior change.

In Table 5.1, we illustrate the balance of informing, asking, and listening that characterizes each of the three styles. The directing style

TABLE 5.1. Examples of Directing, Guiding, and Following Styles with Offenders

Situation	Directing	Guiding	Following
Supervising officer meeting an offender to develop a community management plan	"There are some rules you're going to have to follow. Let's go over them."	"I have here a list of your conditions. Which would you like to start with: treatment groups, finding a job, where you're living, or meeting with me?"	"Why don't you tell me why you're here?"
Meeting with an offender who was 20 minutes late for her last substance abuse treatment group	"You seem to have some trouble getting to group on time. You need to fix that or you're going to get kicked out of group."	"You were late to your last substance abuse group. Let's talk about how group has been going for you."	"How have you been this past week?"
Working through a vocational plan with an offender with little work history	"You don't have much work experience. I have some advice on how you should go about getting a job."	"It sounds like you've wanted to work but have had problems finding a job. What kinds of work have you considered?"	"What kinds of things do you like to do?"

heavily emphasizes informing, or giving the person information and advice, with moderate degrees of asking questions. Within this style, questions serve primarily to gather sufficient information. Little attention is given to active listening. As part of a following style, listening is emphasized most, with questions used sparingly to facilitate the listening process. Providing information or advice is rare. The guiding style uses all three approaches almost equally, as each may be appropriate given the circumstances. The goal is to listen, ask informed questions, and to guide the person toward discussion of pertinent matters without being too directive or forceful. How do we use a guiding style with offenders? Each example demonstrates how one might find the middle ground of a guiding style while working with offenders at various stages of involvement in rehabilitation and reentry. Similarly, Box 5.1 describes this style in a correctional setting, where the offender might have responded far differently had this staff member used a different style.

While MI adopts a largely guiding style, there are times when one would give advice (i.e., directing) or more strongly commit to active listening and reflection (i.e., following). To most effectively use MI, you must remain ever aware of the style of your communication and ensure that it is deliberate, appropriate, and in the spirit of the goals you hope to facilitate in the offender.

BOX 5.1. GUIDING STYLE

Suicide watch units in correctional settings involve the continuous observation of inmates to prevent self-harm. Occasionally, offenders make false claims of suicidal intent, or they feign psychosis, in order to be placed in a segregated, secure unit. Their reasons for this vary. One interaction with inmate Montoya, a young man newly sent to the watch unit, was memorable.

"What brought you to the unit?" I asked, curious.

"I'm hearing voices," Montoya responded.

A lengthier conversation and some clinical observations led me to think that Montoya was not, in fact, suffering from a psychotic disorder. I did not challenge him about that but instead switched to his reasons for wanting to be on the watch unit. "How were things going on your unit before you came here?"

Montoya explained that it was his first time in an adult facility, following years of being in and out of juvenile facilities. He had not yet made any friends or acquaintances on his yard and was struggling to get along with his cellmate.

"It sounds like you have a number of reasons for wanting to be here, instead of there," I reflected. "I imagine, though, that there are some things you miss about being in general population."

He noted that he didn't know he could not have visitation while on the watch unit. He desperately wanted to see his infant daughter—now just starting to talk—and was worried about her being confused by his absence. After talking more about his daughter and his life, he agreed to be discharged from the watch unit. There was no need to confront or even discuss his feigned symptoms of psychosis, and it maintained our relationship for future therapeutic work.

—Adrienne Lindsey, MA, DBH, Arizona State University, Tempe, Arizona

PROBLEMS WITH COMMUNICATION

Developing and maintaining a guiding style is not always easy. And though there are situations in which directing and following styles are appropriate, you may find yourself "stuck" while using them. Common problems with communication style involve using "muscle" or meekness to the exclusion of effective communication, pushing for things to be "just right," or struggling with a sense of balance between influence and control.

Muscle versus Meekness

We use the term "muscle" to convey overuse of a directing style with an offender. Using muscle means providing information and advice, giving orders, or directing a one-sided conversation, incorporating very little of a guiding communication style. In this context, listening is a means to an end, or simply a way of providing a pause for you to compose your thoughts about what to say next. A muscle approach relies on a position of authority to dominate and demand compliance from the offender.

This muscle approach is unlikely to be very effective. No one enjoys being confronted with shortcomings, ordered around without consideration for their thoughts or feelings, or dominated by persons in authority simply because they are in the one-down position. Imagine that you are seeing your physician for a minor physical ailment, and he or she interrupts you, criticizes your weight or diet, gives you a lengthy list of directives to follow, and then strongly admonishes you for asking questions because he or she is the doctor, and you are simply the patient. Most of us would leave such an encounter feeling disempowered, frustrated, possibly humiliated, and certainly angry. This hypothetical physician's use of "muscle" to get his or her point across, even if well intentioned, is likely ineffective. Using this approach with offenders inspires a similar result. They feel diminished, disinterested, and defiant. Thus, using muscle is not only unsuccessful but potentially even counterproductive. It hampers your ability to enhance behavior change.

However, there is danger in going too far in the other direction. A following style does not inevitably connote passivity or weakness, but it has the potential to do so. Overuse of a following style can turn into what has been called "professional dangerousness" (Turnell & Edwards, 1999). This happens in a fairly predictable way: You work hard to gain the other person's trust and engage him or her in treatment, supervision, or other rehabilitation efforts. You become fearful of anything that will send you back to the start or weaken this hard-won rapport. But the person does something wrong that should be addressed, and you feel reluctant to mention it at the risk of losing ground. You find yourself saying, "I won't tell this time, but don't do it again."

Here lies professional dangerousness. Efforts to avoid directiveness and muscle have instead fostered passivity, meekness, and ineffective following. In this case, the pendulum has swung too far to the opposite extreme, and you avoid being directive when perhaps you should be. The hope of building an alliance and meaningfully working together with challenging clients does not necessitate ignoring critical violations of the rules. Believing offenders are worth doing business with is not the same as adopting the easiest way of doing business with them (Turnell & Andrews, 1999).

Finding balance and determining the most effective style to use in any given moment or interaction requires you to carefully monitor your intentions and style in each communication and conversation, recognizing that communication style can and should be flexible at different stages of the process. MI promotes a guiding style, which allows you to incorporate different styles as needed while maintaining a helpful and balanced approach overall.

The Expert Trap

In Chapter 4, we discussed the righting reflex, or the tendency to push back when one meets resistance. We also noted the danger of the expert trap. These are again relevant as we discuss client engagement and communication style. You are likely to encounter resistance when you present yourself as the expert, or the one with the right answers. Much like with Goldilocks's three porridge bowls that were too hot, too cold, and "just right," be on your guard for the idea that you can make everything "just right." This vexing issue arises as you try to avoid styles that are too directive (muscle) or too permissive (professional dangerousness). This dilemma is disguised by good intentions. Most of us truly want to help, which is the primary reason people choose this challenging, and often thankless, work. Helpers have a natural desire to fix what appears wrong. This translates into a desire to change the trajectory of an offender who seems headed in the wrong direction.

Going about this using an overly directive style and efforts to force the offender onto the right path paradoxically pushes the offender further from change. One pushes based on the urge for perfection and the assumption of expertise. Helpers can fall victim to their own innate and natural drive to set things right. You want to stop what might hurt someone, and you think that you have a more objective, correct, and informed way to go about it. So how can it be that what seems like the best thing to do only makes things worse? The reality is that we are not always the experts, nor must everything be "just right." In fact, this "just right" is often not the only or even the best answer. Offender work is highly complex. It is fine for things to remain imperfect (in our view) for a time in order to allow the person adequate space and autonomy to self-determine his or her own needs, rather than try to enforce a different and more directive way. Change is ultimately more meaningful when people come to it on their own, and you have to resist the reflexive and impatient need to get them there faster. In this case, pushing too fast and using directive communication almost guarantees that the process will slow down.

> *Pushing too fast and using directive communication almost guarantees that the process will slow down.*

Understanding Control versus Influence

Another similar problem is learning to use influence rather than control to bring about change. Finding the distinction between influence and control is important. Control is the extent to which one person attempts to regulate or restrain another person or situation, as when the court provides specific orders for a probationer to follow and threatens sanctions for noncompliance (Botelho, 2004). This is an effort to control behavior. There is little choice involved. Control is evidenced by a singular use of the directive style, with little or no inclusion of guiding or following styles. To tell the truth, there are times when we must use control and directive communication to achieve the mission of ensuring safety and social control. A person who represents imminent harm to self or others, for example, requires more directive and at times coercive efforts.

Fortunately, we do not always find ourselves facing such dire circumstances. Once assured that the person is stable or safe, you can turn again toward behavior change. It is unlikely that you can do so through coercion and control. The alternative is *influence*. But what is it? Influence is how you help a person decide whether to change, without coercion or force. MI emphasizes influence rather than control. True and lasting solutions are based on acceptance (i.e., the person recognizes and accepts that the change must occur) rather than shame and condemnation. To influence, you must foster the positive, keeping in mind the differences between using "power with" and "force over" to facilitate change (Hawkins, 1998).

"Power with" is an idea consistent with the spirit of MI. The elements of partnership, acceptance, compassion, and evocation ensure that power is shared, and that the work of change rests with the offender. Again, you work with—not on—the person. The client is ultimately responsible for change, and you use your influence to guide the process and keep it moving forward. Framers of strength-based conceptualizations note that while you may be able to make a person meet with you, listen to what you have to say, or even show up for therapy, *you cannot force them to change* (Ward & Maruna, 2007). Successful treatment and rehabilitation necessitate active acceptance and willing participation from the offender. One can foster these conditions through a guiding style.

"Force over," on the other hand, speaks to control and authority. Whatever benefits it may offer for temporary stabilization or for ensuring compliance, coercive force works against lasting behavior change. Overuse of force exacerbates resistance and noncompliance

> *The client is ultimately responsible for change, and you use your influence to guide the process and keep it moving forward.*

in the long term (Hubble et al., 1999; Miller et al., 1993; Miller & Rollnick, 2002; Tomlin & Richardson, 2004). Offender control has been viewed as a simple problem of math: if there are violations of the law, it is because the consequences weren't punitive enough (Gladwell, 2013). We know that this is not the case. But this mind-set is pervasive and encroaches on our own work, despite what we know about the effectiveness of influence and "power with."

A CLIENT-CENTERED APPROACH: MOVING FROM MUSCLE TO MOTIVATION

A client-centered approach holds that clients possess both the drive and the know-how needed for their own behavior change. Put simply, a client-centered approach is based on the assumptions that the person has the internal resources to improve and is in the best position to resolve his or her own problems. This approach is most associated with its founder, Carl Rogers, a famous counselor and researcher from the 1960s and 1970s. Rogers (1951, 1986) believed that in order for a client to improve, the counselor needed to have a warm and genuine demeanor, with the ultimate goal of understanding the person. This approach prompts a climate in which natural drive and know-how can surface. Motivation is not a fixed trait (like having brown eyes) but a state, and a state that can be influenced through just such an approach.

Rogers often downplayed the use of specific techniques in the work of psychotherapy, believing that too much emphasis on techniques depersonalizes one's work and strips away the uniqueness of the individual person. Instead, he placed greater emphasis on the relationship established between counselor and client, spotlighting the need to be receptive and responsive to each individual person and each moment of the conversation. Any techniques suggested were merely tools to aid listening, acceptance, and understanding.

MI grew from Rogers's influential style. Client-centered work, in its purest form, was somewhat passive. Establishing an engaging climate may not be enough for a person addicted to narcotics, or someone who has repeatedly dropped out of domestic violence treatment. They need more. Initial work with MI concentrated on the technical aspects of the approach (Miller & Rollnick, 1991). Such a focus on techniques was necessary to communicate both what a helper should do and how. However, while persons learning MI may have been able to demonstrate the techniques, too often the spirit of MI was absent (Rollnick & Miller, 1995). It isn't all about the techniques. The helper, or the person facilitating conversations about change, needs to understand and demonstrate a certain "spirit" of relating to clients, as we discussed in Chapter 2. The skills without the spirit are hollow—and significantly less effective. It is akin to hearing a concert where the musicians play all the right notes but with no feeling or interpretation. Since then, Miller and Rollnick (2013) have emphasized that the spirit of MI is more important than the practicalities of techniques or tools. But both are needed. Rogers's client-centered style presents a necessary though not sufficient way of working with offenders for change.

This leads us to an obvious question: *Can you be client-centered in offender work?* After all, there are traditional roles and expectations, and one is reminded that the public will think you're being "soft" on the "bad guys." Add to that what you often hear: "They don't know how to change"; "They don't want to change"; "After what they've done, who cares what they want?"; "It's our job to tell them what to do, not to have them tell us." Pessimistic attitudes like these have turned offender interventions into something that you do "to" them, as offenders are viewed as "deficient, ineffectual, misguided, untrustworthy, possibly dangerous, and almost certain to get into trouble again" (Harris, 2005, p. 328). This obviously runs counter to a client-centered style, where the person is seen as capable and responsible for his or her own life choices, including ways of altering those choices in the future.

This presents a glaring dichotomy. Because offenders have committed harmful acts, we are torn between two conflicting responses: (1) the desire to help them change; and (2) moral condemnation (Ward & Maruna, 2007). The hurt and harm they have caused can repulse us and create so much stress that it overcomes a desire to help. In these instances, customary civility (e.g., shaking hands, using a person's given name) or extending basic respect are considered signs of weakness, or signs that you are willing to accept and condone violent behavior. Intended helpers detach themselves from the offender and begin to view themselves as morally superior. Moral appraisal and judgments that put people into categories provide a strong sense of certitude and control. At the same time, you want them to change. You want them to reach the potential you imagine, though they may not see it themselves. How do you resolve this conflict? And how do you engage in a client-centered way, consistent with the spirit discussed in the preceding chapters?

First, enter the relationship with an offender with an open and curious mind. Practice compassion, acceptance, and empathy. The person knows best what works and what doesn't, and also that they have the capacity for growth and change. And second, keep in mind that we are not so different from one another. Our basic humanity is central to these conversations. There may be parts of the offender's life that you cannot relate to, but there are also most certainly parts that you can. This calls to mind a keynote presentation given by Ted Kaczynski's brother, David, at a 2007 conference of the Forensic Division of the National Association for State Mental Health Program Directors (Kaczynski, 2007). Asked what he thought of his brother, who as the Unabomber killed three people and injured many others, he recalled a story from his childhood. He described his brother as a young boy, despondent and crying after losing his pet. David Kaczynski said that this is how he remembered his brother. He did not try to excuse what his brother did, and was, in fact, responsible for reporting his brother to the authorities. Yet he still saw his brother as a person of worth, with genuine emotions and needs.

Staying within the spirit of MI and a client-centered style involves relating to the parts of the offender that are so much like ourselves, giving them the same space and time that we would hope others give us.

CHAPTER 6

ENGAGING

The Relationship in Practice

I've learned that people will forget what you said, people will forget what you did, but people will never forget how you made them feel.

—MAYA ANGELOU

Working with offenders includes many things, like scheduling, supervision, collaborating with others, procuring necessary resources, and completing the inevitable paperwork. But perhaps the most dominant part of our work involves conversation. We talk with people. This is our greatest advantage, and we must learn flexible and strategic use of the core communication skills that MI offers in order to gain the most from these conversations. In this chapter, we'll discuss five core communication skills that promote client engagement. Though they are used throughout all four processes of MI, such skills are greatly needed as we engage with the offender. To begin, we will discuss open-ended questions, affirmations, reflective listening, and summaries (condensed into the acronym OARS), and review a fifth skill, informing and advising. These skills are critical in helping us move the conversation forward. We want the client to talk with us, and we can influence what they talk about. We use these skills while maintaining the spirit of MI and the client-centered stance that is central to all that we do.

ASKING OPEN-ENDED QUESTIONS

An open-ended question is one that gets the client talking and allows him or her the widest range of possible responses. Such questions prompt offenders to more fully describe themselves or their situations. Open questions call forth their ideas, frame of reference, and self-knowledge. Some examples of open-ended questions include:

"What are your thoughts about drug use?"
"How has the arrest affected your day-to-day life?"
"How do you hope your life might be different 5 years from now?"
"Who in your life offers you support?"
"How can I help you comply with your probation orders?"

In contrast, closed questions are queries that elicit short, clipped responses with very little detail. Ask a client, "Do you drink too much?" and you will receive one of three brief responses: yes, no, or maybe. If it is followed by "Do you realize it was alcohol use that got arrested?" you can expect the offender to feel lectured to and thus begin to shut down. Issue a stream of closed questions—"When did you have your last drink?"; "How much do you drink?"; "Have others told you that you drink too much?"; "Do you feel your drinking is a problem?"; "Have you tried 12-step self-help groups before?"—and you feel engagement slipping away.

How you ask questions shapes the client's response as well as your relationship with him or her. Consider the contrast between these two questions (Berg & Kelly, 2000):

"Did you slap your spouse across the face?"

or

"You must get frustrated with your spouse at times. How do you deal with that frustration?"

Each of these questions elicits a certain type of response. The first is a closed question, fraught with accusation and socially driven judgment. The second involves a statement of empathy or compassion, as well as an open question to understand the offender's interpretation of his or her own behavior. You are far more likely to get helpful information with the second question (open) than the first (closed). Unfortunately, though people are often taught to use open-ended questions, they choose instead to use closed questions because they are "easier," or because there is a perception that they save us time. You want to get to the point. However, for broader purposes, it is far more effective to use open questions, as they leave room for more information and build a more positive and engaged relationship with the offender.

There are variants of closed questions, many of which are likely to damage the relationship you have with an offender client. The first of these is the masquerade question, or a closed question masquerading as an open-ended one. For example, you might ask someone his or her plans following treatment, but frame it in such a way that the person has no choice but to answer as you want them to: "What do you hope to do

> *How you ask questions shapes the client's response as well as your relationship with him or her.*

after treatment?"; "Don't you want to get a job?" Or a multiple-choice question, which starts out as an open question but then backtracks by limiting the response options: "So what are you hoping to do: quit or cut down?" Or instead: "What do you think would be the best approach for you: go to individual therapy, begin group therapy, or try that agency class I mentioned?"

A second type is the rhetorical question, where the question is meant to communicate your own intentions rather than to generate a response from the client. There is a desired answer within the question itself: "Don't you think it would be better for you to . . . ?"; "Isn't your freedom important to you?"; "You didn't really expect that to help you find sobriety, did you?" Each of these questions begs an unstated answer. The offender is caught in an unescapable bind, knowing the "correct" answer but unable to give an answer that he or she truly believes in. These questions and their answers do little to move you forward.

A third kind is the tag question, which can take on a rather sinister tone (Berg & Kelly, 2000). The tag question includes a closed question at the end with an obvious, socially laden answer. Some examples of these: "You drank again, didn't you?"; "You want to be honest, don't you?"; "You didn't attend your treatment group again, did you?" In a way similar to rhetorical questions, the expected or desired response is implied. Such questions also carry judgment, leaving the client little room to disagree, state his or her opinion, or offer explanation. Further, the sometimes accusatory tone of such questions damages the helping relationship and reduces the trust and openness that give you traction in the conversation.

Another form of closed question is the "why" question. Not all "why" questions are closed, and in fact, some are very helpful in evoking client strengths and change talk (discussed further in Chapters 9 and 10). However, some "why" questions are closed in that they are meant to elicit brief, simple facts, leaving little room for exploration. Within these questions you see the righting reflex at work. "Why" questions place blame and force the respondent to use excuses to defend the problem. Imagine your own response to these why questions: "Why did you do that?"; "Why did you go to that party?"; "Why did you hang out with them when you knew they were up to no good?" Many of us would find ourselves bristling at such questions. Though open questions, they provoke defensiveness and imply that the client has done something wrong—knowingly so. Rather than encourage reflection and openness, they breed discord and distrust.

It seems simple enough to identify differences between open and closed questions, and there is the risk of quickly dismissing this core counseling skill as something easily understood and worth skimming over. But take a moment to give them a second look. Think back to your own education, when you displayed how well you knew information by answering questions. Rarely were you expected to ask them. Relatedly, seldom does formal training address how to ask the right questions. It is vital to learn everything you can about the offender to facilitate their self-change process. How do you learn another person's perspective? How do you understand what they value? You ask them in an open-ended way and let them talk (Camp, 2002).

The use of open questions may seem problematic for those who work with offenders. Training often emphasizes or reinforces using a shotgun approach—ask many questions at once in the hope that one will be on target, much like the belief that shooting a burst of pellets from a gun will increase the odds of one finding its mark. However, such an approach weakens the ability to elicit meaningful responses. People are not targets. They will become frustrated, embarrassed, or withdrawn in the face of being peppered with closed questions and are less likely to answer any of them. A second problem arises from the way offender agencies structure their paperwork and methods of intelligence gathering. Frequently, official documentation requires you to gather a great deal of specific information, and too often you may devote your efforts to asking a barrage of questions so that you can fill in the necessary blanks. This costs you a collaborative relationship. While recognizing that such paperwork is required, we would encourage you to think creatively about how to accomplish both goals. Asking open questions and allowing the offender to talk often yields more information than sticking to checklists and mechanistic routine. Try open questions, and you may get most of the answers you needed while gaining a collaborative partnership as well. You can always go back to complete your checkboxes after the offender feels his or her voice has been heard.

Occasionally, getting the offender to talk is not the problem, but rather the more immediate problem is getting him or her to pause and take a breath! Offenders can come in anxious, scared, or angry and engage in pressured speech, talking rapidly and with high emotion. They may become tangential or repeat themselves. The offender is talking, and certainly talking more than you may be, but the content or process is not productive. A lack of back-and-forth dialogue does not allow us to influence positive behavior change. Later we will discuss how affirmations, reflections, and summaries can be paired with open questions to slow them down and return the conversation to a more productive end.

Still, please do not finish this section with the belief that closed questions are wrong or inconsistent with MI. As an interview concludes, for example, one might ask, "Did I miss anything?" Also, during the planning process you might ask, "So is that what you're going to do?" These are productive closed questions. The goal is to evaluate the situation, your role in the moment, the emotional context of the conversation, or immediate goals to decide how to proceed. Often, you will know when it is appropriate to start transitioning to more closed questions or even other parts of the conversation simply because it feels natural to do so.

AFFIRMING

From our discussion of PACE, you will recall the importance of acceptance, empathy, and compassion. These important tenets of the spirit of MI critically inform the next piece of engagement and the second component of OARS: *affirming*. The very idea of an affirmation is one that should be familiar to you. When you seek to understand others, you affirm the truth and basic human worth. In other words, you recognize that others are fellow human beings, worthy simply because of a shared, common humanity. Offenders are no different. Their journey to change is filled with unfamiliar territory, and getting there requires significant vulnerability. Within that journey is a need to affirm their worth and the truth and value of their goals.

Affirmation requires several things of helpers or persons involved in facilitating offender change. First, affirming requires a fundamental respect for the other person. With offenders, it is sometimes challenging to maintain an attitude of respect. After all, there are times when you feel that they do not respect you. It is important though to remember that this is a person who needs help, and that this person is going to have to do the work of change to make it happen. In other words, as much work as you must do to complete paperwork, fulfill requirements of your job, or find ways of engaging the offender, ultimately your work is minimal in comparison with what is expected from the person in front of you. Thus, it is vitally important for you to understand the sacrifices and compromises the offender has to make, as well as maintain respect for his or her autonomy in making life-changing decisions. It will likely be much harder than what you must do in this relationship.

Second, affirming another person's worth requires genuineness. Only pretending that you have concern or see value in another human being violates the tenets of partnership, acceptance, compassion, and accurate empathy. Offenders may be particularly attuned to disingenuousness, as they have been surrounded by it in the form of other offenders, families who may only sporadically show concern or interest, or the stream of staff members and therapists with whom they have previously though only minimally known through their contact with the criminal justice system. They quickly become cynical. Within the embrace of cynicism, they may find it difficult to believe that you are genuine, but when you are able to break through and show it meaningfully and consistently, it forges a stronger relationship. How to do this? Challenge your own assumptions. Think about the following questions:

> "Why did you choose your present career? Was there a part of you that believed you would be helping others? Has that changed?"
> "How often have you found yourself laughing with your clients, knowing that for a moment, it was just something humorous being shared between equals?"
> "Do you have a family member or a friend—maybe a person who you haven't seen or heard from in years—whom you later learned had committed an offense? Does that change your memories of the person, or the kinds of things the two of you had in common?"

Obviously, such questions challenge what many of us have been taught in the context of professional boundaries. The intention is not to reduce necessary professional boundaries. But part of being truly genuine is learning to recognize and appreciate the shared things that make us equals as human beings.

Third, affirming involves being strengths-based. This is certainly an area for improvement in the offender field, which strongly emphasizes deficits, limitations, and risks. It is easy to assume that individual weaknesses are pervasive and indicate larger problems with interpersonal functioning, emotional maturity, or behavioral control. But highlighting deficits or failures does little to promote change. It stigmatizes, discourages, and alienates the offender. It damages the therapeutic alliance. And it runs counter to attempts to affirm worth and humanity. Therefore, affirming requires finding and promoting strengths. You only need look. Your clients are survivors. Many of them have faced abuse, poverty and deprivation, negative influences, limited resources and opportunities, risks to interpersonal safety, and periods of hopelessness and despair. Despite setbacks and poor decisions they have made, they have persevered and are now coming to you with the hope of improving their circumstances. So you must find this survival instinct, bring forth the strengths that have aided them thus far, and ultimately affirm that they are worthy of their own efforts to grow and change.

Affirming involves respect, genuineness, and a focus on strengths. This is all good—provided that you know what to do with it. How do we affirm another person? One may mistakenly think that affirmation is

> *Affirming requires finding and promoting strengths.*

praise, or saying "I'm proud of you" in response to a desired outcome. But praise of this kind can imply an imbalance of power in the relationship, or that you hold authority over the person and can judge his or her actions as right or wrong. Instead, start by acknowledging the effort the person has made, or the positive things he or she has done or attempted to do. Focus on what the person has accomplished: "You made the call and set up the appointment"; "You must feel so good after turning in the application and getting a call right away!"; "Your experience in therapy before really helped you get down to work last week." These examples of affirmation highlight the person's strengths and accomplishments. They provide recognition of effort and worth, and they communicate respect in a genuine way.

Affirmations may take other forms. These range from simple acknowledgments—"I'm glad you were able to come in today"—to more sophisticated conversations that reframe ambivalent feelings or behavior: "This has certainly been a struggle. There are times you don't think you can do it, and you come in today and tell me that it's been 3 days since you even thought about getting high. Wow. That's the longest you've been able to do that in a long time." This affirms the person's motivation and efforts to change without creating a power differential or specific expectation. It also communicates respect and genuineness in the moment. It strengthens the relationship and powerfully reinforces change.

REFLECTING

We briefly introduced reflection in Chapter 3, as a core component of active listening. Reflective listening allows you to check your understanding of what the other person has said. Language is more than just words. It includes context, mannerisms, and unspoken needs or intentions. You may not know with certainty what an offender means or intends to communicate in any given interaction. Because offender agencies use so many idiosyncratic acronyms, conversations may be unintelligible to an outside observer. Even among those who understand the acronyms, consistently inferring correct meaning or intention may be difficult. Communication thus resembles a juggling act. All at once, you are balancing what the speaker means to say, what the speaker actually says, what the listener hears, and what the listener thinks the speaker meant (Gordon, 1970). This is much to juggle at once and calls for listeners to reflect content back to the speaker to ensure that what you heard was in fact what the speaker meant to say. Reflecting allows the speaker to hear it as you did, and to correct it if necessary.

Reflective listening is part skill and part guess. People don't always say exactly what they mean. You listen closely and deliberately and then voice a guess about the meaning of what the offender has said. Things may go awry at any stage of the communication process, as shown in Figure 6.1.

First, the speaker must encode his or her meaning into words, and the selection of the correct words is dependent on how well the speaker understands his or her intention, the speaker's comfort with language, and the extent of the speaker's introspective ability. Next, the listener must hear the words accurately and also interpret their meaning. Reflection is a natural next step, as the listener forms a reasonable guess as to the original meaning and voices it back to the speaker as a statement of fact. Why not just ask, instead of making a reflective statement? When you lapse into rapid-fire questions, it detracts from the sense of a

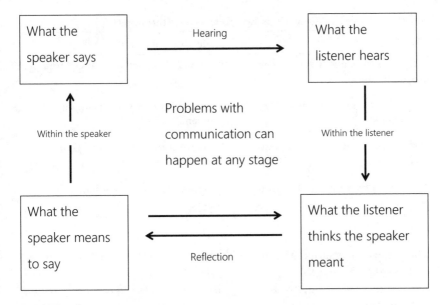

FIGURE 6.1. Reflective listening and the stages of communication. Based on Gordon (1970).

flowing, natural conversation. Question after question makes an interchange seem mechanical and contrived, though the occasional open-ended question provides you with information to reflect. A well-formed reflective statement serves to encourage continued exploration rather than to evoke defensiveness. A question may imply that the person has done something wrong, suggesting that his or her actions or feelings are in question. See for yourself. Consider the differences between the pairs of responses shown in Table 6.1. To hear the difference, you may need to speak them aloud to yourself, as your voice inflection will make them different. You raise your voice at the end of a question but lower it at the end of a statement.

Reflective statements communicate *understanding*. The difference is subtle but significant in offender work. One should remain mindful of a clear power differential (i.e., power over) that can subvert efforts to understand. Questions or prompts to explain behavior can create distance between you and the offender and leave them feeling that you doubt what they say: "Does the staff think I did something wrong?"; "Does my case manager think I shouldn't have felt that way?" Another even more negative outcome would be for the offender stop thinking

TABLE 6.1. Paired Questions and Reflective Statements

Question	Reflective statement
"You're feeling angry that you were placed on probation?"	"You're angry that you were placed on probation."
"You don't think your drinking is a problem?"	"You don't think your drinking is a problem."
"You want to switch out of your treatment group?"	"You want to switch out of your treatment group."
"You don't think you did anything wrong?"	"You don't think you did anything wrong."

about the conversation and instead begin thinking about defending him- or herself.

To practice reflective listening, first *think reflectively*. Fully listening communicates neutrality and openness (see Chapter 3). If your mind is filled with judgment and preconceptions, then there is little room remaining for what the offender would tell you. But even when you think reflectively, communication remains difficult. Statements can have multiple meanings. For example, when an offender client says, "I wish the judge would have been more understanding during my court hearing," there are many different interpretations possible: "I didn't get to explain myself"; "I wish the judge could know how difficult my situation is"; "I was angry at what the judge said during the hearing"; "I was sorry for doing it, and I don't think the judge really understood that"; "I didn't do anything wrong, but the judge acted like it didn't matter"; "I felt the judge was too tough with my sentence—it was so unfair"; "I felt really down and wanted the judge to know that." Dismissing any preconceptions for the moment will help you more clearly see these many options, using reflection to hone in on the one that best describes the client's experience.

How do you use reflection? It is a mistake to simply think of reflection as a mere echo—it is far more than parroting back what the person has just said. Carefully listen and reflect key elements of the exchange (simple reflection), and also infer meaning, or read between the lines to get at what the person is feeling and what they would say next (complex reflection). In Box 6.1 we introduce John, a man on probation for theft associated with his drug use. John has a history of depression and aggressive behavior. Our interviewer could be almost anyone—a probation officer, a clinician providing treatment, or a case manager. For illustrative purposes, every interviewer response demonstrates reflective listening. Notice that many of these reflections move the conversation forward rather than just repeating back what John said. The interviewer reflects what might be the next logical sentence, but does so without leading John or forcing his narrative. This is a skillful form of complex reflection that we call *continuing the paragraph.*

Several things stand out. First, the interviewer does not lecture, chastise, or push for change throughout the exchange. It would have been easy to lapse into lecturing or active problem solving instead of using reflections. This is avoided, however, because the purpose is to help John explore his own experience and wisdom. Reflective listening involves a certain degree of trust that people are the experts on themselves, want to be healthy, and can reach their own conclusions. Second, this skillful dialogue could plausibly be a monologue by John alone. Imagine that the interviewer's comments were uttered by John instead, and the conversation flows easily. The interviewer's reflections finished John's thoughts and prompted him to explore further, almost as if he had said them himself. This natural flow cannot happen if the interviewer inserts questions, advice, disagreement, or disgust. To listen reflectively, you focus on the offender's *own* narrative rather than asserting your understanding of it.

Several issues emerge when you reflectively listen, particularly when you focus on it as a deliberate practice. It may seem unnatural to suddenly pay so much attention to how you listen. As you do, however, you begin to take notice of potential problem areas.

1. *Too many words.* Too often we add words to the beginning of a reflective statement. "What I hear you saying is . . . " and "So it sounds like you're feeling that . . . " are common examples. These are unnecessary phrases and take the focus off of the speaker, putting it on us—the listeners—instead. It is a subtle shift: the focus should be on the person speaking rather than the person listening.

2. *Making an interpretation.* Those new to reflective listening may feel pressure to interpret what the client is saying, particularly when using complex reflective statements. However, reflection is about the views of the speaker, rather than the perceptions of the listener. At this stage of the process, it is reflection rather than interpretation that is important. For example, if an offender said, "I got really mad at my boss yesterday," an interpretation might be "At that moment, your boss was treating you just like your father used to treat you," whereas a reflection

---

BOX 6.1. JOHN'S INTERVIEW USING REFLECTIVE LISTENING

INTERVIEWER: Okay, John . . . positive for marijuana. You told the tech that you had smoked it about 2 days before your urine test.

JOHN: About 3 days before. I made a mistake. I was stressed out, and money was a big part of that. I just freaked out.

INTERVIEWER: Finances have been weighing on you.

JOHN: I mean, we have enough to get by, but we struggle. We are barely making it. I got two kids, a wife, the rent . . . and I worry. I worry about paying the bills.

INTERVIEWER: You were feeling pretty down about yourself, and you're wondering if you can do this.

JOHN: Yeah. I talked to my wife. She said to stick with it. Try to get back on the meds. So I swallowed my pride and went to the doctor. But then it was an ego thing. I don't want to have to take a pill the rest of my life to be normal.

INTERVIEWER: You thought you had some control.

JOHN: Yeah. But I didn't.

INTERVIEWER: The meds are supposed to help you stay clean and sober.

JOHN: The doctor said it would help my mood. It's an antidepressant. And then maybe I wouldn't need the drugs.

INTERVIEWER: You had hoped that the meds would help you think clearer and deal with the stresses in your life, rather than getting high when you feel overwhelmed.

JOHN: Yeah, but why do I see that as a weakness? And my girl, she obviously knew that I had relapsed. I don't know, but I think she's done with me. But I can't help it. I don't feel like I have control anymore.

INTERVIEWER: You're really worried that you're going to lose your family.

JOHN: I can't. I love them.

INTERVIEWER: A life without your family is no life at all.

JOHN: Without her and the kids, I'd be like I was before—selling drugs, pulling guns on people, and thinking that I'm bulletproof.

INTERVIEWER: It's about your family, but ultimately it's about you, too.

JOHN: It's them. It's me. I just don't know.

INTERVIEWER: You're scared that you're not going to be able to get over this, and you're frustrated because you don't know how to fix it.

JOHN: But the pills are supposed to help, you know? It's just that I've never been much for pills. Oh, I think I'm way too cool to need pills. But look at me now. How cool am I?

INTERVIEWER: You don't want to take pills, yet you keep getting high.

JOHN: Yeah, exactly. It doesn't make sense, does it? Maybe it's time stop trying to be cool.

INTERVIEWER: It's time for a change, and the meds might be part of that.

JOHN: I'd say I got nothing to lose, but I do. My wife's about to walk.

INTERVIEWER: It's time for something different.

mirrors back what the offender said, such as "What your boss did yesterday upset you and left you feeling angry."

3. *Agreeing with them rather than reflecting.* We may become gripped by the fear that our attempts at reflective listening could be construed as agreeing with what the offender has said. We are used to challenging or confronting incorrect or unhealthy statements, rather than reflecting them. For example, an offender may state, "I love getting drunk. I work hard, and it's okay to let my hair down after work." We might respond with "You believe it's a reward after a hard day's work." This is a reflection. If we were instead to say, "Nothing wrong with rewarding yourself, right? You deserve it!" it would communicate agreement. There is a difference between the two, and we want to be mindful of what we say. A good reflection mirrors what the person has said but does not condone, reassure, or grant permission. Instead, you express your understanding and recognize the value of the other person's viewpoint, even if you disagree with it.

4. *Reflecting everything back as a question.* Good reflections are like observations of the weather. If you and your coworker are walking into your building from the parking lot in a driving rainstorm, upon reaching the building and shaking off the water, you wouldn't turn to your coworker and ask, "It was really raining?" No! You would definitively state, "It was really raining!" It is a fact that you both know to be true. It is important in providing accurate and meaningful reflection to avoid asking tentatively. Reflections are a clear statement of shared understanding.

5. *Fear of getting it wrong.* What happens if what you reflect back is wrong? Or if you miss an opportunity to provide a good reflection? No one likes to be wrong. We especially don't like to be wrong when it may involve looking foolish or ineffective at our jobs. But what happens when you get it wrong? In our experience, the speaker simply corrects

you and moves on. They may still appreciate that you tried, or that you were listening that closely to what was said. There is no penalty for your mistake. The conversation continues, and you both gained something from it.

This may seem like a great deal of effort. Reflective listening can be hard work at first—harder than the barrage of questions we are accustomed to. However, it will become easier with practice, as is true of most learned skills. Good reflective listening keeps the person talking, exploring, and considering. Once the offender is talking, you can focus on the direction of his or her speech, which will be discussed further in the next two chapters.

SUMMARIES

Until now, we've focused our attention on open-ended questions, affirming the client's worth, and reflection as the bases upon which to build engagement. Now we turn to summaries, or helping bring the conversation together. Summaries are essentially a collection of reflective statements that you pick and bundle together, much like a floral bouquet. Summaries serve several purposes. They condense the client's statements into a manageable and coherent whole. They affirm the client's worth and value, communicating to the speaker that you're listening and want to get it right. They also lead you toward focusing, the next stage of the MI process. Summaries keep the client talking and can also influence *what they talk about*. There are three types of summaries that assist the interviewer.

Collecting Summaries

In this straightforward type of summary, you reflect back what you've heard in a condensed fashion. Sometimes offenders, much like anyone telling his or her story, can become distracted or forget the point they were trying to make. At these times, they can become lost or stalled, and even well-meaning listeners can disrupt the flow or use this as an opportunity to jump in with their own observations. With a collecting summary, however, the goal is to get them back on track without inserting yourself into the conversation any more than is necessary. A collecting summary reorients the speaker and invites him or her to continue. Below, an example:

JOHN: And then I went to my counseling appointment, which went okay, and then . . . and then, I . . . um . . . (*goes silent*).

STAFF: So, John, let me make sure I understand this. You had a decent day at work, and thought your boss might give you more hours, which can help pay your restitution. You found a ride to your counseling appointment, and you were proud that you were able to ask your sister for a ride to make sure you made it to your session on time. You thought the counseling appointment went okay, and that felt good. What else is important to talk about?

Collecting summaries can also help with another issue. Sometimes offenders may divert from a productive conversation and move into an angry or pressured rant, and you struggle with the balance between stopping it and getting back on task versus engagement and maintaining the alliance. The collecting summary can allow for both, as it gives the offender a chance to vent some frustration but also allows you to reflect and move the conversation forward. For example:

"John, wait. John . . . please wait. Just a second. What you're saying is important and I want to make sure I've understood all that you're telling me. You said [condensed summary]. Do I have that right?"

Some offenders have limited cognitive abilities and skills. Others are in crisis and feel emotionally and mentally overwhelmed. Such states may interfere with anyone's capacity to reason and problem-solve. Amidst these scenarios, it is helpful to stop and summarize the important points that have accumulated. Collecting summaries allow the speaker to review and consider what he or she has said in a more integrated fashion. Offenders hear themselves describe their experiences, but then they hear you reflect what they have said in a way that encourages them to continue.

Linking Summaries

While some may only interact with an offender once, others interact with the same offender on many occasions, with relationships spanning weeks, months, or even years. Linking summaries allow you to connect experiences or issues discussed in earlier sessions to the present moment. For example:

> "John, let me see if I've got this right. First it was problems with your counselor yesterday. Then today, you got really mad at your boss. I remember you've also talked about how another boss you had a couple of years ago at your last job did some of the same things. I wonder if your ability to keep it together in spite of your frustration helped you avoid trouble yesterday when you got upset with your counselor."

As this example illustrates, the linking summary draws on strengths and past experiences to bolster coping behavior in the present. Linking summaries are akin to collecting summaries, but with content that has been discussed over time. You selectively bring in past material to help the offender "connect the dots" from what happened then to what is happening now. This additionally helps move the conversation in a productive direction and reinforces past experiences consistent with change.

Transitional Summaries

The transitional summary is used to close a particular topic and shift to something new. They may also assist in moving from one MI process to another, such as moving from engaging to focusing, or evoking to planning. They are also very useful in concluding a topic that has reached its limit:

> "You mentioned how last week's hearing made a big impact on you. Parts of it felt unfair, and a lot of it made you angry. You were especially upset with what the prosecutor said, and now you're feeling pushed into probation supervision. The whole process felt like being dragged through the mud. Before we begin to talk about my role and your supervision, what else would you like to add?"

Note how the speaker reflected what had presumably been said at various points throughout the session and then moved to transition into the next part of the conversation. A transitional summary often begins with an orienting statement, or one that announces that you're about to tie things together before changing directions. The substance of the summary is a collecting summary, highlighting the two sides of the offender's ambivalence about change, or emphasizing important feelings or beliefs that will play a role in the offender's decision making. But it does not end there. The final piece is the *key question,* which invites clients to transition from talking about *why* they are considering change to focusing on *how* they see themselves incorporating new behaviors. This key question, and how the person responds to it, is very important. Some examples: "How do you see yourself taking the next step in accomplishing your goal?"; "What do you think the next step is?"; "With where you're at, what should you focus on now?" Answers to these questions tell us whether or not the offender is ready, if there are early indicators of change occurring, and what may be needed to formulate a plan. The key question serves as a guide in moving the conversation forward.

INFORMING AND ADVISING

While the OARS skills are crucial for engaging the offender and maintaining the conversation as you move into other stages of MI, there still remains the question of when to give information and advice. The reality is that our jobs often require us to provide specific pieces of information, or at least to ensure that clients know certain rules. Does MI proscribe such efforts? After all, we've noted several times the need to minimize an overly directive, advice-giving style. Does this mean giving it up entirely? And won't it make you seem soft or weak in comparison with standard practice in offender agencies? If the answer to these common concerns was a solid yes, many would not want to use MI with offenders. But the answers are far more complex and should be considered more thoroughly.

Informing and advising are the last of the core communication tools we review in this chapter. It seems straightforward—offenders need advice, and you have it. Why not give it to them? But a more important question from an MI perspective is: *Why won't they take it?* Using a motivational style raises the odds that the offender not only *hears* the advice but also *heeds* it. To inform and advise while still engaging with the offender, there are two important components to understand. First, offer advice with permission. And second, work to understand the offender's perspective and position before approaching him or her with information or advice.

Advice with Permission

Our first consideration is how to give advice without being directive. No one responds well to orders, particularly when the relationship is still new and trust has not yet been fully established. So when do you offer advice?

One such time is when the offender asks for it. Sometimes a person will directly ask, "What should I do?" Or maybe "What do you think is best?" Here, you have clearly been given permission. But still, tread carefully and avoid a directive style. Elicit ideas from the offender first, and then perhaps use those as a point upon which to further the discussion: "I have some ideas I can give you, but I'd like to hear what ideas you have before I go into that." Another alternative is to offer more than one option, thus maintaining the importance of respect and autonomy: "You have several options here. I'll go over them with you and you can decide what may work best for you."

Another time is when you ask permission to give advice. Perhaps the conversation has come to a natural point to discuss options, or the offender seems open to your ideas following your reflections and apt summaries of the situation. Asking for permission allows clients to still say no, while alerting them that you are being respectful of their choices. Some examples of how we may do this include: "Would it be okay if I gave you some information about . . . ?"; "I know that many others I've worked with have also been frustrated by this—would you like to hear about some things they have done to make it better?" You may also preface your advice with permission to disagree. A person who is upset and angry may not give permission, but if you still feel it is important to introduce the idea, you can give advice with the understanding that they do not have to take it: "This may or may not work for you, but one thing you might think about is . . . ."

At this point, the goal is to engage the client. Information and advice that are part of focusing or planning will be addressed further in subsequent chapters. For now, any efforts to provide information should be those meant to further elicit the client's willingness, or to communicate appreciation of his or her circumstances and needs.

Understanding Perspective

Engaging involves working to understand the offender's situation and what may be most helpful. It is easy to overestimate how much information and advice is necessary. To be sure, offenders may expect you to have answers. Yet they already possess a wealth of relevant information. No one knows them better than they know themselves, so it is crucial to start with assessing what they do know. From this, you can determine what they know, what they've tried, and what they view as the root of the problem. It helps very little to offer them advice that they already know, or to suggest something they've already (unsuccessfully) tried. You want to avoid the trap of offering a suggestion and hearing back why it won't work. Instead, try to understand the offender's perspective, and use that to generate additional ideas. See Table 6.2 for several examples.

We close this section on information and advice with a reminder about offender autonomy. Though offenders face forthcoming consequences for choices that violate court orders, the freedom to choose always remains with the client. They know the consequences without us telling them. Even in moments where it is appropriate to inform and advise, the client still maintains autonomy and choice. Within offender systems, it can be described as a three-step process.

1. When an offender balks or disagrees with a court order or program rule, remind the offender of his or her choice in the matter: "John, you say you don't want to go to this alcohol class, even though it's one of your court orders, and that is your choice."
2. List the consequences in a neutral manner. There is no need to frighten or bully the offender into compliance. Keep your tone conversational; you are simply providing facts: "I've seen this happen before. If you choose not to go, I can tell you that _____ will happen."
3. End by reaffirming that the choice is the offender's alone: "But it's still your decision to make, John. You can take the consequence if you'd rather. No one can make you do this."

You want them to hear more than just your words. Remember that the melody is sometimes just as—or more—important than the lyrics.

TABLE 6.2. Examples of Less versus More Effective Ways of Providing Information or Advice, Using the Offender's Perspective

Less effective	More effective
"Couldn't you borrow your mother's car?"	"So you've said it's very important for you to keep your meetings. How are you going to make that happen?"
"What about that job at a fast-food restaurant?"	"A fast-food place might be one option, but I'm wondering what else you've thought of?"
"The next time you get angry, make sure you count to 10 before acting."	"When you think about times where you've been able to manage your anger, what things have worked for you?"

The tone is always important as you inform or advise. You do not want to come across to the offender as coercive, or as simply imposing another rule to follow. Pressure undermines internal motivation by making someone feel manipulated. Thus, remember your role in the process— the client is the expert. You are there to facilitate growth and behavioral change. To do so, you listen, affirm, reflect, and summarize key points to take the offender further along in the process. Doing so makes the relationship stronger, and the client is more than a passive recipient of your plan. The client is engaged, and the next step is to focus on what lies ahead.

CHAPTER 7

FOCUSING AND PREPARING FOR CHANGE

Everything can be taken from a man but one thing: the last of
the human freedoms—to choose one's attitude in any given set
of circumstances, to choose one's own way.
—VIKTOR FRANKL

In the practice of MI, we start with engagement. It's a crucial piece of the
puzzle, but not the only piece. The offender needs to be engaged for the
conversation to develop, but the conversation must gain direction or it
will wander and stagnate. This is why we focus—to find a sense of direction or purpose as we move forward. Offenders enter the conversation
with a unique set of values. The values are theirs—individually shaped
by their experiences, beliefs, relationships, emotions, and the like—and
they continually shape the offender's goals and ambitions. The conversation is ever changing, and it is important for us to have a sense of direction as we advance.

In this chapter, we will discuss the process of focusing, while Chapter 8 will describe the mechanics and application of this stage of MI.
First, we will examine who's involved in setting the focus. This includes
who decides where we go from here, as well as how the pathways differ
depending on the various goals and viewpoints of the people involved.
Second, we will describe the role of ethics and values in focusing the conversation. When working with offenders, it is a difficult thing to say that
the goals of the system are not paramount (e.g., don't reoffend, don't
hurt people further). Thus, it is important for you to take time to think
about your own values and how these influence the process of focusing

the conversation. Finally, we will delve into ambivalence and the process of developing discrepancy—two crucial components of focusing that we must negotiate successfully if our work is to progress.

THE PURPOSE OF THE CONVERSATION

Focusing is a fluid and changing process. As conversations about change evolve over time, you will see changes in focus—necessary changes—that are dependent on natural changes in offenders' lives. Offenders' discussions of their goals for behavior change are impacted by their hopes, fears, expectations, and concerns. For example, consider the brief monologue from John, our offender client introduced in Chapter 6, presented in Box 7.1. Here, John describes what he hopes to get out of his court-ordered treatment.

John's statements highlight the need for focusing. Creating a list of his goals illustrates why John has struggled with finding a place to start.

- Control mood more effectively.
- Be compliant with psychiatric medications.
- Participate more in treatment.
- Make a better life for his children.
- Doesn't want his children to repeat his mistakes.
- Feel more in control.
- Make his own decisions.

These are all important goals, and some are stated more clearly than others. Yet even those that linger beneath the surface remain important. John expects that treatment will help him and that once he commits, he will stay committed. Such complexity illustrates the challenge of this next stage of MI, where John must identify one or more paths, balance his needs, and select the most appropriate course.

Sources of Focus

John's perspective—or that of any offender client—is only one piece of finding the right focus. John has already given us several points to explore further. But the client is only one source of direction. Another source is the agency or setting where you work. If you're working with John, you are all too aware of other requirements set by the court. And part of your job might be to ensure that all requirements are met, not

---

BOX 7.1. JOHN DESCRIBES HIS CHANGE GOALS

"I mean, I'm not happy that the judge is making me go to treatment. It's not that I don't need it, but I would feel better if I had a choice. But well, I guess that doesn't matter. Now I've got to go. But it's not like I haven't thought about therapy before. I have had some meds before to help with my mood, and they did help, but I just didn't take them seriously. Thought I could do it on my own if I could just get myself together. I need help with my drinking. I don't like feeling so out of control. I used to just do it when I felt bad, but then I seemed to need it all the time. Then when that wasn't working as well anymore, or when my girl got onto me for drinking too much and losing it, then I took some drugs. Thought I could have more control over that. I've been to treatment before, and it didn't work for me. But I just didn't do it right. I don't think I ever really bought into what they were saying. It was too much to think I had to change it all at once. But I want a better life for myself, and for my family, you know? I don't want my kids to grow up like I did, with a drunk for a dad who was never there. And I don't want them to grow up and do the same things I'm doing. I think it's all just a matter of 'walking the walk,' right? I just have to commit to it and the rest will come."

---

only the one that the client chooses. Different settings vary widely in the latitude they give offenders in determining their own path. Even if you can't give them more latitude yourself, you can always give them a greater voice in how or why they comply with requirements. There may be consequences, but the decision remains with the offender.

You also have your own expectations and input into what the focus should be. Your expertise and experience can also guide the conversation, even as you recognize that clients are the experts on themselves. We reconcile this difference by knowing that our own experiences can fill gaps in knowledge or supply examples of how others have accomplished similar goals (with the client's permission to give advice, as noted in Chapter 6). There is also the possibility that you might have worked with John (or someone very similar to him) before. This can limit your view of what he can or should accomplish, and this can lead to the expert trap (Chapter 4). Instead, continue to use accurate empathy and curiosity about the offender's world, recognizing that even if you've been there before, things may have changed since the last visit. Even new failures have merit; we often learn more from failure than success.

For John, there are also societal goals to consider. Don't reoffend. Get your life together. Treat others well. Be a productive member of society. There is no need to articulate these goals to John—*he knows them.* How he forms his goals and develops a change agenda is dependent on his culture and his investment in the goals and expectations of that culture. Thus, the purpose of the conversation from an agency or societal perspective is implicit. Let's not waste time stating what is already known.

How We Communicate

In Chapter 5, we introduced the three styles of communication: directing, guiding, and following. Directing is an authoritative, definitive style. We are directive when we are simply telling others what to do. Following, on the other hand, has little focus and requires us to follow wherever the client takes us. Guiding is the style most evident in the MI manner of focusing. The client is talking, engaged in the conversation. The conversation needs continued direction, and we guide the client toward that direction without stating what it should be. The purpose, then, of a guiding style during this phase of MI is to allow the client room to explore while still maintaining a coherent picture of the tasks that lie before us.

THE VALUES AND ETHICS OF FOCUSING

The skill of focusing can be achieved but takes practice. It involves uncertainty and shared control. You will also face ethical dilemmas, or situations in which your own values or views may emerge and give you pause. It is important to be aware of this. The goal of MI is not for you to adopt new values or ethical standards. At the same time, however, you are not the most important person in the conversation. Your work to find focus for the offender honors both your values and his or her needs.

Do No Harm

The phrase "Do no harm" is crucial to the helping professions and to work with offenders. As agents of offender systems, your work is premised on the assumption that you protect people from harm. Your clients may have caused harm to self or others through their illegal behaviors. You enter with a mind-set of preventing future harm, regardless of your role within the system. Therefore, it can be challenging to move your focus from working to prevent crime to working to improve the offender's behavior and lifestyle. Change makes the person better. Change also prevents crime. Are the goals really all that different? Still, there are times when your values push you to emphasize prevention and avoiding harm, though adherence to the spirit of MI urges you to focus on the goals most meaningful to the offender. Keep in mind that you can accomplish prevention and harm reduction through building a strong relationship with the offender. Focus on relevant offender goals and they will, in the end, result in greater behavior change and more harm prevention than punishment or a caustic attitude.

Do What Is Good

A second concern goes beyond "do no harm" and instead emphasizes doing what is good. Can you promote the good, given the sometimes overwhelming need for avoiding harm? The simple answer is *of course,* though it may not seem so clear from the outset. A fear is that helping or "doing good" overlooks the harm that has already occurred or that could recur in the future. Yet change for the good promotes both goals. You are also not being easy on offenders by working for what is good. Their work will still be difficult and involve significant change. Doing what is good is best not only for the offender who develops his or her goals, but for victims, communities, and others who are impacted by crime. Focusing on goals and needed changes involves a balance of "do no harm" and "do good" that runs throughout the work of MI.

Autonomy

Though we have already discussed autonomy in the context of the spirit of MI and engaging the client, autonomy is critical to focusing as well. Autonomy reminds us that as we go forth to find direction, the client maintains his or her voice in the process. The client has an important stake in determining the goals of change. Autonomy means many things, but in the process of focusing it means that the client retains important choices. This is consistent with a guiding style of listening. Your role is to listen, learn, and be strategic in highlighting the client's available options. Returning to John's discussion in Box 7.1, we see several potential topics for him to address in treatment. He mentions a need to control his mood, his drinking, and his use of drugs. He also wants a better life for his children, and he wants to create a better life for himself. Most importantly, John wants

> *Your role is to listen, learn, and be strategic in highlighting the client's available options.*

to commit to treatment and make changes in his life. All of these are good goals. Pursuing any of them would satisfy the problems or needs noted by the court or other involved agencies while still maintaining John's autonomy and respecting his choice. John will make a stronger commitment to these goals than ones devised without his input.

Justice

Working for justice is not the difficult part. We work with offenders out of a sense of justice for past and future victims, and to help offenders reenter the community with the best possible outcome. Instead, the challenge is in determining whose justice is paramount. The mission of offender agencies often harkens to societal justice, or justice for specific victims. But in contrast with the early beginnings of the criminal justice system—when offenders were brutally punished without regard for their humanity—there is now a call for justice or fairness in how offenders are treated as well. MI is also concerned with the rights and respect given to the client. During the engaging process, you embody the spirit of MI and hear what clients have to say. It would seem wrong to suddenly stop doing that as you begin to focus the discussion. Justice, then, is embodied in focusing as well. You listen with fairness, knowing that some goals may be more or less important than others. This is what focusing is about. Clients have the opportunity to consider outcomes, and you guide them in such a way as to help them identify those that are most important and meaningful. This begs a critical question—do you want to be right, or do you want to be successful?

Your values are important. They help to make you an effective listener, and to keep you centered on the goal of behavior change. Yet when you find that your values conflict with those of the client, or when you are unable to balance the goals of offender change and important systemic priorities, it can be helpful to reflect on the ultimate purpose of MI, and your role in the larger process. You are having a conversation with an offender who needs your help and support in finding direction as he or she moves forward toward change.

AMBIVALENCE

At the heart of ambivalence is conflict—feeling both positively and negatively about the same thing at the same time. Or instead, holding mixed views about a subject without a clear resolution in sight. This state of ambivalence causes discomfort, and this discomfort is at its worst when it is time to make a decision. The ambivalent person is caught between knowing a decision must be made and being unable to choose between alternatives. It is then that the person becomes stuck.

Why do people get stuck? That is, why do people lapse into a state of indecision, seemingly wallowing in conflict between two or more alternatives? In many cases, particularly those involving offenders, the correct path seems quite clear to those of us viewing it from the outside. It appears easy to select the preferred alternative. But the person remains ambivalent. There is typically more than one way to reach a goal and more than one goal that has appeal. Most people are ambivalent about change. They know they need to change—their pain and trouble tells them that. Yet their problematic behavior has benefits they're not sure they want to (or can) live without. Ambivalence takes many forms: Can versus can't, should versus shouldn't, and want to versus don't want to. Life balances precariously on a decisional seesaw, and *it is a common human experience*. In fact, this teetering is so ordinary that it is considered a natural part of the change process (DiClemente, 2003; Engle & Arkowitz, 2006).

During the conversations, you hear offenders voice reasons for change, describe efforts to change, and express commitment to change—and you jump on this as if it were a life raft. This leaves you disappointed, angry, and betrayed when they fail to live up to those commitments, or engage in the same problematic behavior that they were just regretting. Because just as people can voice a commitment to change, they also voice allegiance to their past, fearing the unknown. Contemplating change—and all that comes with it—can be intimidating. The offender becomes stuck, moving neither toward nor away from change, wavering indefinitely with no clear sense of direction or finality.

An integrated perspective on ambivalence involves several important elements (Engle & Arkowitz, 2006). First, the person must believe change is necessary, or hold a desire to change. In the case of offenders, you may not always be privy to this knowledge; they may not immediately discuss the part of them that wants to change in a deep and meaningful way. Anyone would feel anxious and vulnerable considering an important change. Second, the person must believe that change, in some way, will be beneficial. Some past experiences with change are loaded with pain and failure to the point where offenders are no longer sure that change is good. Third, the person must see strategies that facilitate change, which could come from any number of sources, as available or accessible. This could include treatment or other guided intervention, prior experience, or self-directed learning and practice. Fourth, though the person understands how to use these strategies, he or she does not use them. Conversations about change likely reveal barriers to using change strategies, as well as limits in motivation and resources. And finally, the person feels negatively as a result of his or her failure to use available strategies for change. In short, this model of ambivalence posits that a person feels and understands the need to change, believes it will be beneficial, knows that there are available solutions, yet fails to use them and feels badly as a result.

Of course, not everyone is ambivalent. Some people need to change but see no reason for it, or believe it will not benefit them to change at the present time. Their behaviors have caused harm to themselves or others, but they are committed to maintaining the status quo. Such persons are rare. More often, it appears that a person has little interest in change only because you have not yet gained their trust or listened sufficiently. You discover ambivalence by listening. Still, there are some with no interest in change. For these offenders, the goal is to create or develop ambivalence, so that they can move forward in their discussion of change. (This is addressed further in Chapter 8.)

Yet the majority of offenders are stuck or ambivalent. People who have violated the law are aware of the downside of their behavior. People who have had problems with drug use often know that they should quit using. People with anger issues can list the consequences of their verbal or physical tirades. At the same time, people can describe how good it felt to avoid using drugs or hurting others, or to have healthy and appropriate relationships. So why don't they just change? It should be an easy decision. But herein lies the challenge. Other motives and rewards conflict with doing the right thing, even outweighing the desire to avoid punishment or the rewards of prosocial behavior. Again, ambivalence is both wanting and not wanting the same thing.

People can remain stuck in ambivalence for a long time, moving back and forth between choices and never reaching a conclusion. Persistent ambivalence has a familiar pattern: think of a reason to change, think of a reason not to change, and then stop thinking about it. The path out of ambivalence requires choosing a direction, following it, and continuously moving in the chosen direction. MI, and focusing specifically, helps the offender choose a direction, guiding the person in selecting one that will lead to meaningful and rehabilitative change.

Not every path is the one *you* would choose. The challenge is to avoid becoming stuck yourself. Too often, you become trapped in blame or judgment of the offender's ambivalence. This is best demonstrated through statements that begin with "You would think . . . . " For example:

"You would think that having your children taken away and put in emergency foster care would be enough to remove a woman's ambivalence about drug use and would compel her to cooperate with child protective services."

Or:

"You would think that time spent in prison, with its deprivation and day-to-day misery, would dissuade a man from reoffending and stop him from even considering another crime after he gets out."

People are quite sensitive when discussing topics about which they feel ambivalent, in part because they fear judgment, but also because they have likely had these same discussions internally. The righting reflex and an overly directive style of communication set up an oppositional pattern of conversation. With MI, you instead use a guiding style and curiosity to find ambivalence. Consider the benefits that could be realized if people who work with offenders universally believed that people have a side that wants to change as well as a side that does not. This change alone would revolutionize the field.

DISCREPANCY

No one feels encouraged when another person is stuck or ambivalent. However, understanding that most offenders are already ambivalent about their behavior becomes a great advantage in our work. Once you are aware that ambivalence is present, the next task is to develop discrepancy between where the offender is now and where he or she would like to be. Here is where you find the focus of the conversation. As the offender reflects on the status quo—being under supervision, being incarcerated or hospitalized, or subject to the orders of one or more agencies—the goal is for the person to see a future that is somehow different, as well as desired. Awareness of that discrepancy will spark his or her motivation.

Exploring Values and Goals

We often lament that the offender just isn't motivated. But wait—are you sure? To say someone is unmotivated is akin to saying the person doesn't have a personality. Everyone has a personality, even if it is one we find difficult or very much unlike our own. This is also true with motivation. All offenders have motivation, but it might be that they're not motivated in the way you would prefer. Change happens in the lives of our offenders all the time. Greek philosopher Heraclitus (535–475 B.C.) is known for postulating that change is central in our universe, noting that everything changes, and that the only constant is a state of change. Motivation and goals are subject to this same process of change. At times, what motivates us may be basic—as fundamental as our need for food or sleep. But when such basic human motivations are satisfied, we pursue higher goals.

Offenders also have higher goals and values that emerge once other needs have been met. Understanding these core goals and values leads you to better appreciate their frame of reference. What are their hopes and desires? How do they understand their meaning and purpose in life? What do they stand for, live for, and aspire to? You may be tempted to think that some only live for crime, or that their aspirations are to make easy money, or even that their purpose in life is to satisfy their own selfish desires. Harboring this view runs counter to the spirit of MI that was discussed in Chapter 2. While we can understand the pessimism, such thinking gets us nowhere. Seeing offenders in new ways more effectively helps them. Peele, Brodsky, and Arnold (1991) capture this idea in describing people struggling with serious drug addictions: "More often than not people rise to the occasion when they are given positive options. People typically strive to set their own lives straight, and given time usually succeed. Nearly all people have values that are incompatible with their addictions" (pp. 162–163). Offenders have values incompatible with their illegal behaviors.

Why explore values and goals? Because when you understand what people value you are in touch with *what motivates them*. What are the offender's long-term goals? How does the person want his or her life to be different a year from now, 5 years from now? You understand problems by looking from past to present, but you find solutions by looking from present to future. Exploring potential life goals also broadens a person's perspective, lifting his or her eyes from current troubles to a better future. Understanding a client's values and goals is another way to promote engagement and provide a solid foundation for a working alliance (Chapters 2 and 5). You may not always agree with the values being expressed, but it is important to convey acceptance and respect. Honoring human worth in tandem with the offender's most valued ambitions not only improves the relationship but lays the foundation for change to begin. From these values, you are poised to work with discrepancy.

Exploring Discrepancy

A person's life goals are an important source of motivation for change. Why? Because aspirations and values guide behavior. When a person's behavior falls short of how he or she wants to be, or when behavior contradicts core values, it can motivate someone in the direction of behavior change. This highlights the presence of discrepancy, or a difference between where one is and where one would like to be. People become aware of these discrepancies when invited to reflect on their values and actions within a safe, nonjudgmental atmosphere. Such self-examination and self-awareness can be uncomfortable, of course, and your task is to help the offender sit with discrepancy without reverting to defensiveness. Listening, reflecting, and using the tools to be explained in coming chapters are all excellent strategies for doing this.

The spirit of MI discourages a confrontational style. Yet we acknowledge that self-confrontation in this process is inevitable and, in fact, desirable. To confront means to come face to face. What we want to occur isn't confrontation between you and the offender, but instead the struggle within the person. The client's dilemma provides the momentum needed for change. For example:

- Jim wants to keep drinking, despite his recent DUI and court-ordered counseling. With only 2 years to go before he retires, he faces losing his job and worse—losing his hard-won retirement pension.
- Alice is not sure she wants to stop using marijuana, as it helps her with her anxiety and panic attacks. But now she faces the threat of Child Protective Services keeping her newborn in foster care until she can complete a drug evaluation and pass her urine tests.

You help the offender examine and explore this discrepancy on his or her own to enable this momentum to surface. Your role is to negotiate that realization in an affirming, supportive, and compassionate way. After all, even the best of us have discrepancies in our lives. We can easily relate to the sense of disappointment, shame, and frustration that the offender feels when falling short of important goals. The goal here is to create a climate in which offenders can come face to face with themselves and reflect upon on behaviors, attitudes, and values. This also honors the offender's inherent worth and autonomy, trusting that they want to move away from their problems and instead move toward more positive ways of living.

Exploring discrepancy necessarily causes some evaluation of the source—is it your discrepancy, or theirs? Obviously, criminal behavior is not aligned with your own goals and values, nor those of our society and legal systems. The focus must be discrepancy between the offender's behavior and his or her goals and values. Your goals and values, while present, are not the source of discrepancy. Unless the problem behavior is in conflict with something that the *offender* cares for and values, there is no basis for MI to be effective. In short, if there is no discrepancy, MI cannot successfully guide meaningful change. So does that mean you should force the offender to see the discrepancy, or create one? No. You are striving to foster intrinsic motivation for change. The offender must truly believe that change will serve him or her by satisfying important values or goals.

There are certainly ways that people can either coerce or manipulate a person into making necessary changes, as in the case of overly directive supervision officers using the muscle approach, or family members or therapists using coercive ultimatums to push a person to engage in substance abuse treatment or marital counseling. But these approaches, while embraced by persons who favor confrontation or pressured compliance, fail to produce lasting and meaningful change. They also violate the person's autonomy and push successful rehabilitation further away.

> *The focus must be discrepancy between the offender's behavior and his or her goals and values.*

MI, by virtue of its reliance on discrepancy between current behavior and deeply held intrinsic values, cannot work in violation of a person's autonomy. When the conversation influences a person to commit to healthy behavior change, it is because the anticipated change is ultimately consistent with important personal goals and values. It is not because of unique persuasive abilities, and most certainly not as the result of coercion. Compliance is not change. Know, though, that engaging and focusing do not require the removal of consequences that the court has already assessed, nor do they suggest suspending future penalties for noncompliance or reoffending. In some way, contingent problems, penalties, or simple hassles certainly can increase discrepancy. It is not, however, your role to create problems in order to foster discrepancy. It is likely that these contingencies are already in place. Those skilled in using MI can help the offender reflect on his or her own values, goals, and behavior in order to bring them face-to-face with discrepancy. The purpose is to develop a meaningful change plan—not to increase offend-ers' anxiety and create additional consequences simply because change has not yet occurred.

What do you do with discrepancies once you have identified them? Merely knowing that the person has goals and values that could motivate meaningful change is not enough to make it happen. There are strategies that help find focus. Knowing where your own values lie, the nature of the client's ambivalence, and the importance of discrepancy helps you focus on facilitating client change.

CHAPTER 8

FOCUSING IN PRACTICE

If a man does not know to what port he is steering, no wind is
favorable to him.
— SENECA

To find purpose in the conversation, we must have focus. Exploring and understanding the client's values brings focus. Diving into ambivalence brings focus. Developing discrepancy, or further contrasting "you're here" from "but you want to be there" brings focus. Much like making finely tuned adjustments to a camera lens, you go back and forth in the conversation to find the point at which the client sees his or her path more clearly. Your role in this process is complex. If you truly remain in the mind-set and heart-set of MI, you are both the lens through which the client can see his or her problem more clearly, as well as the means of adjusting the lens to bring light and precision to the image the client wants to see. A particular challenge in this stage of MI is to share control—to remember that you are a guide who facilitates change, rather than a general who orders it.

Here we delve deeper into the practice of focusing. This includes ways to elicit discussions about values and strengths that will free the client from the stickiness of ambivalence and move toward behavior change. It is also the use of strategies to sharpen the conversation and assign priorities. It further includes the consideration of equipoise, or trying to maintain as much neutrality as is warranted. Finally, we will additionally note strategies for resolving important differences in prioritizing goals. As we review each of these important components of focusing, we remind the reader of the importance of a guiding style and the value of the client-centered relationship to keep you on course.

ELICITING DISCUSSION
ABOUT VALUES AND STRENGTHS

Sometimes the client begins the conversation with a clear sense of direction about what needs to change. This may become readily apparent as early as engagement work and developing the alliance. When the client has a clear focus from the outset, exploring the pros and cons of each possible destination seems counterproductive and unnecessary. Doing so seems to put the engine in reverse, causing the conversation to stagnate. However, it is still important to gain the client's permission to move ahead in that direction before beginning the work of evoking (see Chapters 9 and 10). It would be unfortunate to miss opportunities for discussing ambivalence that could help solidify the client's motivation. In such cases, it is not that ambivalence is absent. It is likely that the client has been stuck in ambivalence before, or he or she would have already made the change without your help. Instead, the client has already resolved some of the ambivalence, and the balance has tipped in the direction of change as you have worked to engage and understand the client's world. Another possibility is that the client's stated goal is disingenuous; offenders may know what to say to move things along. In this circumstance, continuing to discuss ambivalence may highlight the offender's lack of genuine commitment to change, which lends itself to further work and also may accomplish some of the important work of change regardless.

However, in many cases, the client remains ambivalent about one or more options, or alternatively is unclear as to what to do next. For these instances, exploring the client's values and strengths will help him or her focus and clarify goals. In MI, you do this primarily through two methods: agenda mapping and orienting. Agenda mapping is of great use when the client has multiple goals, conflicts between goals, or significant ambivalence, whereas orienting is best for the client who is unable to develop a defined vision of the change or changes that should occur. Let us examine these methods in greater detail.

Agenda Mapping

Before beginning any journey, it is helpful to consult a map. The map provides you with more than just a picture of where you want to go. The map illustrates both where you are and where you want to be (i.e., discrepancy), as well as alternate routes or even alternate destinations (i.e., ambivalence). In a conversation about change, it is similarly helpful to have a map, or an agenda, to guide you. Agenda mapping is a method that allows us to step back and take a look at where we're going and how we could get there. It is less about the change itself and more about how to have the conversation. Consider the following example.

> "John, I'm wondering if it would be a good idea for us to step back for a minute and look at where we are. You have talked about many things you'd like to do differently. You'd like to get your mood under control. You'd like to drink less. You want to stay away from drugs this time. You'd like to have a better relationship with your wife and kids. And you also want to have a better sense of being in control of your life. That's a lot to take on at once, and it feels pretty overwhelming right now. I'd like to look at each of these and figure out what makes the most sense to start with. How does that sound to you?"

Note how the case manager provides a summary of John's previous concerns and also reflects his feelings of being overwhelmed and ambivalent. Within the summary, the case manager also asks permission to go ahead and put these things on an agenda, so that he and John both have a sense of where subsequent conversations will lead. The agenda is certainly complex, and John will need to think carefully about each of his options in order to choose a path. This represents the first component of agenda mapping, when you and the client *structure the agenda*. The purpose is to identify what the options are, rather than to examine each of them in depth. John provided a number of potential options. For other clients, the options may not be as clearly defined, or may still need some additional work. Additionally, there may be options that the client has not yet considered. Thus, another way of going about structuring the agenda would be to say:

> "John, we've covered a lot of different topics and directions you could go in. We need to think about where to start first. I also have some ideas to think about—things that were raised in your last court hearing. But I want to start with you. Would it be okay for us to go ahead and talk about where to begin?"

This is a similar starting point, but one that has not yet honed in on major concerns and therefore provides greater flexibility. It leaves room for the idea that additional concerns from the court may be on the agenda, even if John has not yet explicitly mentioned these. It is important to agree to an overview of what will be discussed, and to make sure that both you and the offender client are on the same page before moving forward.

The next step is to *consider the available destinations*. In our first example above, John has already provided a number of options. In the second example, John has not yet provided detailed options, or perhaps has made statements about "needing to change" or "needing to be in control of himself." At this point, it may be helpful to use the OARS skills you have already learned—ask open questions, affirm the client's views, reflect what the client has said, and summarize the options you have heard thus far. You can also encourage the client to consider other options that have not already been mentioned, or to judiciously offer suggestions or theoretical examples. As with other information and advice (see Chapter 6), it is best to use this latter strategy with the client's permission, and in the context of considering options unknown or unfamiliar to the client.

Once the options are on the table, so to speak, it is time to *zoom in*. Until now, you and the client have been working on creating and looking over the map of the agenda from afar. You have not yet narrowed in on any particular topics, nor have you thoroughly exhausted all of the possibilities. During the process of targeting specific points on the map and zooming in on them, you and the client will transition from exploring every option or scenario to narrowing the options. Here, we target those most immediately relevant and desirable. You need not narrow down the agenda to only one path. Rather, you want to help the client move from considering all of the options to considering those that may have the greatest impact on behavior change.

This can be far more difficult than it sounds, however. In the context of offender services, what the client sees as most relevant may not reflect the priorities of the court or criminal justice system. A client like John, for example, may zoom in on options like improving his relationship with his wife and children, taking his mood medications, and finding stable employment. In the broader picture, these are all good options. All of them will likely assist him in making important positive changes. However, the court will expect regular reports related to his alcohol and drug use, as well as his participation in relevant treatment programming. While the goals John wants to target are important, the court will care little for them if he continues to use alcohol and drugs against court orders.

Agenda mapping, considering available options, and zooming in on topics of greatest importance are shared efforts between you and your client. You maintain a guiding presence in the conversation, but not a controlling one. Being too directive, judgmental, or critical of the offender's goals can compromise all of your hard work at client engagement and establishing a working relationship. Being too passive—overlooking court mandates or required treatment elements merely to maintain the relationship and the client's willingness to keep talking—is not recommended either. You must find the balance. Use a following style (Chapter 5), remembering that the easiest or more automatic way is not always the most productive way. Let us consider a guiding style as depicted in Box 8.1, where John is reviewing his options with his case manager, mapping the agenda and zooming in on what he needs to address.

BOX 8.1. AGENDA MAPPING AND ZOOMING IN WITH JOHN

CASE MANAGER: Okay, John. You have a lot of things weighing on your mind as you think about what you want to do next. We've talked about family, your arrests, your history of depression, and some problems with finances and finding a job.

JOHN: Yeah. It's a lot, really. I don't even know where to start.

CASE MANAGER: I can see that it would be a problem. Looking at all of it, what do you think about the most?

JOHN: Probably the stuff with my family. I mean, I don't want my kids to end up doing the same things I did. And I know my wife has just about had it. I can't imagine losing her.

CASE MANAGER: Your family is very important to you.

JOHN: Yeah. The most important. So maybe I should think about doing something for them instead of myself.

CASE MANAGER: What do you think they would want you to do?

JOHN: Oh, man. I hadn't thought of that. They would want me to stay out of jail. I think that's what would hurt them most . . . me being gone.

CASE MANAGER: Ah, I see. Because they're so important to you, you want to do what's best for them. Being there for them might be best. Staying out of jail is a way to do that. How do you stay out of jail?

JOHN: Quit drinking and drugging. Ha—like that's easy. But that's what it would have to be.

CASE MANAGER: That's what the court told you.

JOHN: Yeah. I hate thinking that that's what it comes down to, but yeah. And it would be better for my family.

CASE MANAGER: You have other things that are priorities. But that one is also a priority. And they all get you to the same goal, really.

JOHN: They do. So let's go there.

Look at what the case manager does. With John's mention of his family, the case manager knows that John has several priorities, of which complying with court orders may not be ranked highest. All of us would agree that John's priorities are certainly important, and one would want him to make these life improvements while also following his court requirements. But how do you interject? The support of a healthy family is a protective factor that lower's John's risk of reoffending. Yet John was arrested for drinking and drug use, and the court doesn't value family togetherness with the same immediacy as passing a drug test or staying sober. The case manager skillfully asks, "What do you think they would want you to do?," knowing that John will turn to his problems with the law and his need to stay with his family. Connecting the value that John places on his family with his court orders is a way of zooming in. A connection is made between valuing his family and keeping the court off his back—all without becoming too demanding (directive style) or too passive (following style).

But what if John had not provided that opening? How else might the case manager have referenced court orders without too being directive or wandering off topic? Perhaps something as simple as: "I know your family is important. What else is important to you? You have court orders, and I worry about you going back to jail. Is that something we can talk about?" This combination of partnership, accurate empathy, compassion, and reflection maintains the relationship and also gives credence to the priorities of offender systems. John doesn't have to agree that the court orders are more important than his family, but family and sobriety are framed in such a way that he can see the case manager is maintaining an eye on the bigger picture while valuing John's own goals as well. A prominent purpose is to help John realize a win–win scenario.

Sometimes the process of agenda mapping may be facilitated through the use of visual aids (Miller & Rollnick, 2013), in the same way a real map of the terrain is used to graphically depict direction. A diagram of important goals, associated values, or even outcomes can serve as a reminder of where the conversation may go. This practice also offers the benefit of getting back on track if the conversation reaches a stopping point or becomes tangential.

Orienting

Thus far, we have reviewed strategies for finding focus when the client has multiple ideas or goals to be discussed. But what if the client doesn't have a clear sense of where he or she needs to go? What if you (or the client) cannot identify primary goals? Let us return to John for a moment. Imagine if he were to begin the conversation in that state. He and his case manager have built some rapport, but the conversation begins to feel unproductive. Take a look at Box 8.2 to see what results.

One open question—*what would it look like if things were fixed?*—gets the case manager and John to the same place John started in the agenda mapping example in Box 8.1. However, this latter conversation didn't start that way, as John was initially berating himself for his poor choices and making vague statements about feeling out of control. The tone of the discussion provided little insight into potential outcomes, goals, or even values that might inform further conversations, and John's statements led down a path of self-criticism and hopelessness about his ability to change. In a situation like this, it is important to orient the client and guide him or her to more productive discussion.

One must first *understand the situation*. This comes from the process of engaging clients and moving into their world to understand it as they do (Chapter 3). The listener uses his or her knowledge of the client's world, and orienting may call for expanding that knowledge. Continue

---

BOX 8.2. ORIENTING IN A DIFFUSE CONVERSATION

CASE MANAGER: Okay, John. It seems like we've covered a lot of ground in these past few discussions. Where do you think we need to go now?

JOHN: I don't know. I just want to get myself together.

CASE MANAGER: You have felt really out of control. Time to stop the merry-go-round and collect yourself for a bit.

JOHN: Right! But I don't even know where to begin. I screw everything up. Every time I try to change, it fails. I'm just a failure.

CASE MANAGER: You're really angry at yourself, too. You let your family down.

JOHN: I know. And I need to fix it, if that's even possible at this point.

CASE MANAGER: What would it look like if things were "fixed"?

JOHN: I'd feel better. Happier, I mean. And more in control of myself. I'd have a better relationship with my wife. We wouldn't argue all the time. We wouldn't fight over money. Or my drinking. I wouldn't need to drink to feel better. And my kids wouldn't have to see us fight. My kids would be happier, too. I don't know that they're unhappy now, but they sure would be if I went to jail.

CASE MANAGER: Okay. That sounds like a good place for us to start.

to use OARS to help you more firmly grasp where the client is in the moment, and to go deeper into the current ambivalence. However, in doing so, resist the temptation to zoom in too quickly on one piece of the picture at the expense of others. The situation is always complex, or the client would easily be able to build the picture without help. Thus, you wait until the whole picture has emerged before mapping the agenda from the various components that make up that picture.

Once the situation is more clearly understood, continue orienting through *precision tuning,* or focusing, the broader picture. This involves a combination of moving from the broader picture to more specific issues within the picture, and then generating and testing hypotheses about the goals and values expressed. This is illustrated in Box 8.3, where John's conversation with his case manager in Box 8.2 is expanded.

In this segment of the conversation, the case manager tests the water and briefly explores several options in greater detail. John identifies goals that were not immediately apparent, as the conversation reveals more about his situation and the order in which some of his problems have occurred. This may have been unknown to the case manager until this point, and it changes the direction of the conversation. We now begin to understand one of the causes of some of John's troubles—or at least the starting snowball that rolled downhill to create a larger one—and we can more firmly view the landscape in which John lives. He indicates some willingness to address his issues, which may be useful in initiating and sustaining other changes later on. During this stage, he is not yet ready to formulate a plan, but the listener can help orient John so that a future plan is tenable.

Again, among the options of directing, guiding, or following, a guiding style is needed. You continue with strategies already learned, like offering a menu, asking permission before soliciting advice, and reflecting selected statements that move toward the client's stated goals. You do so without being directive, as this inserts too much of our own agenda into the conversation. Explore and respect the client's ambivalence, recognizing that if change were simply that easy, the offender would have already been well on the way to behavior change without your help.

CLARIFYING THE GOALS

You have your map, or at least a rough sketch, of the surrounding terrain, if you can answer these questions.

BOX 8.3. ORIENTING IN A DIFFUSE CONVERSATION, CONTINUED

CASE MANAGER: We have a few things that you've identified as important. Your emotional well-being, or your mood. Your relationship with your wife and kids, and whether or not they are happy. Learning to control yourself without drinking or drugs, and staying out of jail. Does that sound about right?

JOHN: Yeah. It's a lot, though, isn't it?

CASE MANAGER: Yes, it is. I won't lie. But these situations are never easy.

JOHN: Right. But where to start! What do you think?

CASE MANAGER: Well, let's see. I want to know more about what you think of these things. Let's start with your mood. You want to be happier.

JOHN: Well, yeah. Doesn't everybody? I guess I've been unhappy for a long time though. Lots of stress. I haven't been able to hold a job very well in the past, and that's affected us financially. Then we fight about money, and the kids get upset hearing us fight. I drink so that I don't have to deal with all of it. I just zone out that way.

CASE MANAGER: Your mood then is affected by all of the stress, rather than the unhappiness being the source of the problem.

JOHN: Maybe. It does seem like the stress and other stuff came first, though I know the mood part is what makes me drink and use drugs more. I was never very good about taking my meds, so I probably didn't really give them a chance to work.

CASE MANAGER: Do you think they might have worked, had you taken them correctly?

JOHN: Maybe. It's something I could try.

CASE MANAGER: That's one thing then. This is the first time you've mentioned having problems getting a job.

JOHN: That's always been an issue. No job, no money.

CASE MANAGER: What kinds of work have you done?

JOHN: Little bit of everything. But I quit school too early, and I never went back for my GED. And I don't know what I really like doing. I always just take whatever's available.

CASE MANAGER: Maybe then you'd like to look at some options there, too.

JOHN: I'd like that.

- Do you have a visual representation of the client's major values and goals?
- Have you gotten a better idea of where the ambivalence lies?
- Are the goals clear, and agreed upon by both the listener and the offender?

- Is there clear discrepancy between where the client is and where he or she wants to be?
- Has that discrepancy been fully discussed?
- Has your discussion of their discrepancy widened the gap between "here" and "there"?

If you are able to answer "yes" to these questions, then you might be ready to move on to evoking. But maybe there were problem areas along the way, or perhaps you want to continue testing your hypotheses a bit further before moving ahead. And with offenders, the problem might not be identifying their goals but reconciling those with what you know must be addressed from the court or other agency requirements. We will address this important point later in this chapter. But even if goals have been roughly identified, jumping forward too quickly can result in greater ambivalence. As with quicksand, the more the client struggles with ambivalence, the more firmly and deeply he or she will become mired in indecision. The solution for helping an offender become unstuck from their ambivalence is to accept it and work with both sides rather than trying to overcome it by force. This is a particular trap to avoid as you clarify goals. Let us consider several others.

Choosing from Too Many Topics

Offenders often present with complex needs. This complexity may, at times, feel hopeless. Their problems are interrelated, interdependent, and often time sensitive. Added to that is pressure on us to prioritize orders from the court or expectations from an offender service agency. Agenda mapping is crucial for this problematic aspect of focusing with offenders. Being aware of the many pressures and priorities can help people make informed choices about where to begin. They are less likely to forget or overlook a high-priority need when it is obvious from a list of options, or to minimize it when they realize the reach of its impact. It may be appropriate to explicitly state or reflect the difficulty of choosing from so many available options or outcomes. This is what the offender is already thinking and demonstrates the accurate empathy and partnership that MI promotes.

Getting Unstuck

It is easy to become mired in a certain topic, or to reach a point where the conversation is no longer moving in a productive direction. This can happen for any number of reasons—perhaps the client is rehashing the same issues again and again, or you both feel a need to stay with the targets that have been prescribed by the court or a particular agency, or the client is continually bringing up new concerns before old ones have been sufficiently discussed. It eventually becomes clear that this is not helpful, and that you are, in fact, losing focus rather than moving closer to it.

There are several potential solutions. In the same way that agenda mapping allows you to step outside the conversation and talk about the conversation, we can also be fairly direct about feeling stuck. You can assess how the client feels about the direction the two of you have taken and continue from there. Another tactic may be to shorten the agenda mapping process by providing a brief summary of where you are and then ask the client to pick the top-priority issues. When you and the client feel pressured to remain on a certain topic past its point of usefulness because of an obligation to the court (e.g., talking about an offense, reviewing conditions of supervision), a simple acknowledgment of how much both of you feel a need to stick with that topic, despite other topics that need be addressed, can perhaps help you move along without feeling like court orders haven't been given their due.

Raising a Difficult Topic

As you work with offenders, it may be very much on your mind that some things remain to be discussed. A violent offense. A drug problem. Sexual misbehavior. Power differentials that lie beyond your control. Sometimes offender clients are open to discussing these matters with little introduction, or you have sufficiently built the therapeutic alliance as to make these matters less sensitive in the moment. However, other times you feel the client slipping away as you approach these issues, or the client avoids or minimizes the importance of these topics altogether.

Discussing these difficult topics requires an engaged offender and a strong alliance. If your level of engagement with the client is not strong enough, it may be time to return to the relationship and use OARS to allow the two of you to rejoin each other, again reaching a "shoulder to shoulder" relationship. Also, the client's autonomy is still relevant. The client always has a choice about whether or not to discuss a particular issue. This does not, however, mean that you are somehow prohibited from mentioning a specified topic, or skillfully inserting it when it relates to the client's values. However, MI makes us aware that forcing the offender to talk about it means we have fallen into the premature focus trap (Chapter 4).

Asking permission is a powerful tool. For example:

> "You've been talking a lot about everything you've lost as a result of being arrested, and how you don't want to get into trouble again, and all that you need to work on to do that. I think that's a wonderful start. I also wonder, though, about some of the things you've mentioned that could cause you problems. Things you haven't been arrested for—like dealing drugs—but that also might need to be discussed. How would you feel about us getting to that at some point, too?"

In such an exchange, several goals are accomplished. The listener provides a summary of the offender's story, including consequences of being arrested, potential goals, and areas where work needs to be done. Also, the listener asks for permission to explore something that the offender has also mentioned but that hasn't resulted in legal action. This is certainly sensitive, as there are many times when an offender only wants to address those topics most directly related to his or her current legal troubles or court orders. For this individual, dealing drugs is a concern, but not one that may have been listed as a point of intervention. Asking permission, or asking how the offender feels about bringing that into the conversation later, highlights the importance of the concern without being too forceful or directive. The listener has also refrained from placing it on the immediate agenda. For most offenders, the answer may be a simple "sure."

Asking permission is a powerful tool.

Clarifying Your Role

People who work with offenders must negotiate the power of the court, criminal justice system, and agencies that is embedded in their roles. Nowhere is the phrase "wearing two hats" more appropriate than with offender work. This becomes most apparent (and at times, most uncomfortable) during focusing, when you are prioritizing areas of change. It begins with an honest explanation of the duality of your role—you have a responsibility to an agency or system, but you also act as a helper for the offender. Now, as the conversation progresses and priorities are named as a part of agenda mapping, you may find it useful to describe your role and responsibilities in terms of the various options.

Remember, however, that despite the alliance, engagement, or efforts at accurate empathy, there is still a felt power differential between you and your offender client. Rather than viewing this power as a tool of force, remember that when used appropriately, it can be used to change the trajectory of a person's life, bringing forth positive changes that radiate from the person to the larger community. Using a power differential to achieve your own goals, or simply using your authority to push harder for what you think will work, can cause parallel harm.

WHEN GOALS DON'T MATCH: IS THERE ROOM FOR NEUTRALITY?

In their most recent discussion of MI, Miller and Rollnick (2013) devote several chapters to discussion of neutrality, equipoise, and our degree of obligation to be directional in working with persons whose behavior has caused harm to others. They raise the question of whether or not we can or should be neutral when addressing harmful behaviors. This speaks directly to work with offenders.

People who work with offenders see things differently from the average public citizen. Regardless of agency, specific job title, or even training and experiences, agents of offender systems know that offenders are more than the offenses they have committed. The general public may think of someone as a sex offender, a drug dealer, or a gang member. From this viewpoint, a person is little more than his or her worst behavior. However, those who work with offenders every day become familiar with other aspects of their lives. This includes the offenses, of course, but also the struggles with family, stress, mental and physical health problems, poverty and job pressures, self-esteem, and moments of success or important values. The person is more than the behavior, though the offenders' harmful behaviors still remain vital in the process of rehabilitation and reentry.

From this perspective, where do your own priorities lie as you have these conversations with offenders? Society and its emphasis on harm—the broad purpose of your work with offenders—may not take into account other priorities that the offender faces on a more frequent basis. Is it appropriate to approach neutrality in these situations? Can we have equipoise, or a dispassionate balance of risks and benefits of certain goals, when working with persons who have harmed others?

The simple answer is *yes*. Consider, for example, this list of three issues that indicate when MI may be most useful, and that also illustrate why neutrality is so vitally important.

1. *When the goal is an observable change in behavior.* MI is a way of being with the client that increases motivation related to change. If the goal is educating, providing information, or gathering information, MI is less applicable than basic listening or other skills.

2. *When the person is resistant, angry, or reluctant to change.* Some believe that MI works best with cooperative clients, but that for challenging clients, a tough and directive approach is best. This latter approach is value laden and assumes that neutrality is undesirable. The research, however, suggests the opposite. Cooperative clients may benefit from a variety of styles or approaches, whereas reluctant or angry clients benefit most from a guiding, balanced, MI style.

3. *When the listener is able to separate him- or herself from the client's attitude, choices, or the ultimate consequences of the client's behavior.* As you likely know, the first step in working successfully with a challenging client is to separate yourself from the client's own choices and behaviors. Though you are quite willing and able to assist the person through referrals, advice, or assistance, there must be a clear understanding that it is the client's responsibility to take action. Likewise, choices that result in negative consequences rest with the client, and you cannot take responsibility for them.

This third issue—separating oneself from the client's choices—can prove to be a delicate matter. Miller and Rollnick (2013) make the point that certain behaviors necessitate attention, thus shaping the process of focusing. They suggest that certain behaviors or treatment needs are so imperative that they may cause the interviewer to set MI aside for the moment in order to ensure safety or reduce harm. For example, when a person is imminently suicidal, or a violent offender has identified a potential victim and is actively planning an offense, true neutrality is prohibited. The topic of conversation and immediate needs are clear, though one can easily remain in the spirit of MI while addressing these concerns. But these scenarios notwithstanding, there are other situations in which one continues with the process of focusing. A decision about whether to accept job #1 or job #2, a decision about attending couple counseling or leaving an unhappy relationship, or a decision about whether or not to file for disability benefits—all of which may be relevant in your work with offenders—are those that provoke less visceral or value-driven reactions than other decisions regarding behavior change.

Relatedly, there are times when the offense is the highest priority. Perhaps this decision is driven by risk, severity of harm, or the offender's own level of concern. At other times, the offense may fall in line after other critical priorities, like suicidal ideation, homelessness, living in dangerous conditions, or other substantial concerns. One makes these decisions fluidly as the conversation evolves. This constant evolution of priorities informs your role in the focusing process.

There are dilemmas on several levels. First, what do you do when there is a clear, nonneutral issue that the client has failed to prioritize? Or when there is significant risk of harm (or harm that is ongoing), and the client is unwilling to consider that as an option during agenda mapping or focusing as a whole? As we have indicated, there are times when you step outside the practice of MI and do what is necessary to keep people safe. That is a separate process. You still address suicidality, other forms of imminent and serious harm to self or others, or similar matters that cannot be ignored. You reach such decisions through your own values, training, and professional ethics. In these instances, it is necessary to become transparent and make your priorities known. This prevents any feelings of deception or duplicity, and it is possible then to return to MI once safety has been assured.

A second scenario is more difficult. Perhaps there are several important priorities that the offender has listed as part of the potential agenda, but those indicated as highest priorities are not related to court orders or your specific role. You feel a need to address these areas, or you might be remiss in meeting your job responsibilities. Still, you want to respect client autonomy and maintain rapport. What do you do? A first step is making your commitments and role responsibilities known. See an example of this below.

"I find myself in a bit of a bind here. You have a court order to participate in anger management and substance abuse counseling. As we've discussed, it's clear that a high priority for you is finding a job and getting your kids back. You really want to feel more stability in your life. At the same time, you have been through treatment before. So even though your orders say that you have to go to treatment again, you don't feel it's necessary. This is where I have a bit of a struggle myself. You see, I'm supposed to report to the court about your progress in treatment. So it makes it hard for me to really get on board with not going to treatment, or focusing on something else and forgetting about treatment. I'm not saying that you have to do what I want—you can accept the consequences we've discussed. It's still your choice. Yet, I'm wondering if we can keep the court off your back?"

Note the important elements of that exchange. The supervising agent presents the court's side while still affirming the importance of the client's other goals. There remains an inherent, underlying respect for the client's autonomy, as well as a demonstration of respect for the goals and concerns of the court. Making such a commitment known may result in further conversation and perhaps openness to reconsider other options that may be more directly related to participation in the required elements of treatment.

Continue to explore the client's ambivalence, allowing yourself to gain a stronger understanding of the client's thought processes and priorities. As the client maps the agenda for discussion, the various options presented will be pursued in turn, with an acknowledgment of the two sides to his or her ambivalence about change. It is possible, however, that there may be differences in opinion over priorities because the client remains too ambivalent regarding a high-need area.

> *There remains an inherent, underlying respect for the client's autonomy, as well as a demonstration of respect for the goals and concerns of the court.*

It then becomes your responsibility to continue the conversation about the ambivalence, seeking to widen the gap of discrepancy (i.e., where they are vs. where they want to be) and allow the client to reevaluate the importance of various goals. Establishing values, linking the overlooked goal to the client's other, more important life goals, and even discussing the pros and cons of varying sides of ambivalence can all be useful in this process.

Finally, acknowledge the client's right to make choices, even if you feel they are bad ones. You can continue to remain neutral or balanced when the goal is not life threatening, even though the client's decision may compromise his or her reentry success. Again, make your commitments and responsibilities known, with the offender retaining the choice to make his or her own decision. As you move beyond focusing and into evoking and planning, the client may return to other goals. The outcome may not satisfy you, but again, it is not your outcome. It remains the client's. Becoming impatient and trying to force the client toward your goals is not a shortcut; rather, it is like putting the car in reverse and hitting the gas pedal.

CONCLUSIONS AND NEXT STEPS

Focusing involves a back-and-forth exchange of ideas. You map the agenda, explore ambivalence and discrepancy, and come to a shared decision regarding important areas of focus for future conversation. This lays the foundation for the next process of MI—evoking. Once you know the goals, you can evoke talk that supports the goal of change and also examine talk that sustains the status quo, as it gives us further insight into important ambivalence and barriers to change. You additionally seek to elicit strengths that will facilitate the difficult work of change. Focusing has been a crucial step in this transition between building a relationship and establishing a basis for change. We now move forward to evoking that which will build lasting behavior change.

CHAPTER 9

EVOKING

Moving toward Change

> If you do not change direction, you may end up where you
> are heading.
>
> —LAO TZU

Engaging is about developing a collaborative partnership. Focusing means finding your destination and orienting toward it. Next is *evoking*, which continues the dialogue about why the client is motivated to change. Evoking involves calling forth the person's experience of the struggle for change. You want to evoke change talk, or parts of the conversation that lend support to behavior change. You also want to evoke motivation, hope, confidence, and strength. The ultimate goal is to evoke what leads to a reasonable and effective plan for change. This is a great deal to accomplish within the course of a few conversations, or even a few minutes of conversation, but it can be done.

In this chapter, we introduce ideas central to the process of evoking. This includes defining change talk versus sustain talk, recognizing these important components of client speech, reviewing the roles of ambivalence and discrepancy, and discussing some of the unique challenges of evoking with offender clients. Throughout, we will continue with our hypothetical offender, John, as well as examples from our colleagues who work with offenders in a variety of settings. In Chapter 10 we describe practical strategies for addressing change versus sustain talk, as well as how to evoke motivation, hope, and strength. But first, let us build a foundation for our evoking practice.

CHANGE TALK VERSUS SUSTAIN TALK

In MI—and particularly in evoking—we are particularly concerned with two primary categories of talk. The first of these is change talk, or any talk that supports change. The opposite of this is sustain talk, which favors the status quo. For offenders, the status quo could be any number of things that have been difficult to change, including substance abuse, maladaptive relationships, or engaging in illegal behaviors. The terms "change talk" and "sustain talk" denote the differing facets of ambivalence. A part of the person is motivated to change, while another part either does not want to or simply does not know how. It is important to recognize both.

There are two primary types of change talk (Miller & Rollnick, 2013). The first of these is preparatory change talk, or statements that suggest motivations for change. These are called preparatory because they indicate preparation for change or early consideration of change but lack the strength of commitment that says change will likely happen. If you were to imagine change as a hill or mountain, preparatory change talk is the trip toward the summit. It is sometimes a struggle, and sometimes a pleasant climb. But it is uphill. It is possible to roll backward, become tired, or stall on a plateau. But gaining ground toward the summit certainly gets one closer to subsequent change. There are four types of preparatory talk—desire, ability, reason, and need—which we will collectively refer to using the acronym DARN. Each indicates something different about the speaker's level of willingness and readiness to change and should be identifiable as the speaker describes his or her motivation.

> *If you were to imagine change as a hill or mountain, preparatory change talk is the trip toward the summit.*

Desire

One can easily think of why offenders would desire change: Negative, punitive sanctions for wrongful behavior. Unhappiness with the status quo. Feeling out of control, or sucked into the chaos of maladaptive relationships and behaviors. You hear the desire in the following kinds of statements:

"I want to stay out of trouble."
"I would like to feel more in control of myself."

"I wish I could get clean and stay away from drugs."
"I hope things get better for me and my family."

The desire to change is a valuable, though not critically necessary, aspect of change. It signals possibility in continuing the conversation—something for you to grasp as you move forward. However, people can still change in the absence of an overt desire to do so simply by developing new behaviors or new patterns. This is evident from many theories of behavioral change and practice with offenders, as institutions and risk management protocols are often predicated on external controls to elicit change. For example, an alcohol-dependent offender who is incarcerated or hospitalized may have no desire to go without drink, but finds him- or herself able to adjust to life without drinking in an environment where drinking is impossible. This represents change without desire but may only reflect compliance with rules rather than lasting behavior change. Take away the rules, and change may vanish as well.

There are those offenders who see no problem with their behaviors. Still, it is likely that they have some desire to change—it may simply be that what they would like to change is not yet evident, or is not what we would most like to see them address in their lives. At times, the desire may be an internal drive to repair damaged relationships or follow the orders of the court, or a yearning for trust. These are still something to work with, allowing you to continue the conversation and evoke talk in support of change.

Ability

Statements like "I can" or "I could" indicate that the offender realizes an actual or perceived ability to successfully change. Ability is a necessary though fluctuating condition of change talk. It is quite difficult to feel motivated if you think change is completely out of reach. Offenders in particular may suffer from barriers to recognizing ability. Past failures, lack of skills, lack of resources, and lack of positive models are all understandable obstacles that impair an offender's confidence in his or her ability to change. Offenders may also see their conditions of release or supervision as limiting their success, and in some ways, they are right. Again, a lack of resources and limited experience with alternatives are practical realities for many offenders.

Accurate empathy is crucial. Understanding the offender's world allows you to relate to and anticipate his or her unique barriers but also recognize hidden talents or abilities that evoking can nurture. Fortunately, preparatory change talk that centers on ability can be inspired or motivated by a skilled listener who recognizes and highlights the individual's strengths. For an example, see Box 9.1, where John and his case manager discuss his history of attempts to change. This exchange illustrates how early glimmers of change talk can be used to strengthen John's confidence in his abilities and evoke mobilizing change talk (a process that will be further discussed in Chapter 10).

Reason

Offenders have heard—repeatedly—why they should change. These messages come in the form of well-meaning advice as well as criticism, originating from the court, offender agencies, family members, employers or teachers, and society as a whole. Telling them why they should be different is only repeating what they have heard already from many people in their lives. Is it fair then to expect that telling them the same thing now will somehow prompt them to change? Hardly. Doing so will probably add you to the long list of others who have used a directive style to lecture the offender about the importance of change. It overlooks the fact that the offender already knows reasons to change: *Being in trouble with the law has consequences: losing family and friends; facing stigma and societal disdain; losing income or employment opportunities; feeling low self-worth, disappointment, or self-criticism; dealing with depression or anxiety about the future; knowing that change means a better life.* There are many more. Our hypothetical offender, John, has already voiced several reasons for change. He wants a better relationship with his wife. He wants a better life for his kids. He wants to feel better about himself and feel less depressed. He also knows that following the orders of the court will help him complete his probation.

Reasons are certainly important. A person who sees no reason to change is unlikely to successfully do so, or to maintain any meaningful change over time. However, reasons are not the only ingredient in the recipe for change. An offender may be well aware of all the reasons—and even voice them convincingly—but lack other components that will help him or her move from preparatory change talk to actual steps toward change. The risk is that when you hear the offender voice reasons, you think, "Finally! They've got it! Now we can really get to work." And then you push forward too soon, missing critical opportunities for evoking other forms of change talk or developing a richer understanding of ambivalence and sources of sustain talk. This impulse stems from the various interviewing traps discussed in earlier chapters, which can more firmly entrench the offender in arguments against the very changes he

---

BOX 9.1. EVOKING CHANGE TALK AND ABILITY WITH JOHN

JOHN: I mean, I want to do things differently than I am now. [preparatory change talk: desire]

CASE MANAGER: You want to make some changes. [simple reflection]

JOHN: Right! Except that I always screw things up. [sustain talk]

CASE MANAGER: It's hard to know where to begin. [complex reflection]

JOHN: I can make little changes, you know? [preparatory change talk: ability]

CASE MANAGER: You've done it before. [affirmation]

JOHN: Yeah, like when I quit smoking for almost a year. I just took it 1 day at a time, like they said in treatment. I made it a whole day without a smoke, and then 2 days, and then a week, and then a month. Kept going like that for a while. [past success with change]

CASE MANAGER: You took it slowly. That worked well for you. [complex reflection]

JOHN: Now it seems like there's so much to do. It's hard to take that one step at a time. Maybe I just can't do it. [sustain talk] But still, if I just look at each thing separately, it might work. I think I can do it if I just don't get overwhelmed by it all at once. Like each thing has to be done one at a time. I know I can do it then. [preparatory change talk: ability]

CASE MANAGER: Well, yes. On the one hand, you know you have a lot that you want to do differently in your life. And it will make your life better. On the other hand, it's a lot of work. It's hard work, and sometimes you feel defeated. At the same time, it's like when you quit smoking for a year. You took it a little bit at a time, and you didn't worry so much about the bigger picture for that moment. It worked! You were able to stop smoking for a whole year—something you never thought you could do. Looking at your goals now, what do you think you could change? [summary, affirmation, and evoking mobilizing change talk]

---

or she knows are needed. The task, therefore, is to not prioritize reasons for change over other forms of change talk, or to assume that they negate sustain talk. Reasons represent a part of the larger whole.

Need

The offender may also emphasize the need to change. This is evidenced by statements such as "I need to . . . ," "I have to . . . ," or even "I've got to change." These statements emphasize an urgent need for things to be different. They communicate something other than a reason (i.e., the "why" of change) or a plan (i.e., the "how" of change). Need remains informative by itself, as it gives the listener an indication of change's importance to the offender. Hearing desire (*I'd like to*) is still fundamentally different from hearing need (*I have to*).

What underlies need? It may be intertwined with other forms of preparatory change talk. The importance of reasons, for example, can influence felt need. How much a person wants or desires something different colors how much they perceive the need for change. Even ability plays a role. Though it may seem that an offender can perceive need regardless of ability, one who sees change as completely out of reach may begin to rationalize a lack of need. For example, a person in great need of treatment but who has repeatedly failed in the past may say, "I'm fine without treatment. I'm not very good at it, and it's not like it's made a difference for me." Need and ability may be intricately intertwined for some offenders.

Offenders may also acknowledge external pressures, repeated experiences with others telling them what to do, or logical understanding that their behaviors have consequences. Such logical understanding may not directly translate to a deep-seated, felt need or motivation to change. In other words, offenders can recognize and state a need for change without truly buying into it. Sometimes you worry that they are simply telling us what we want to hear. That does happen. But at the same time, you want to take it at face value in the context of the larger story and continue to explore. Even instances of seemingly superficial change talk can lead to meaningful conversation. See, for example, a brief exchange between John and his case manager in Box 9.2, and note how the conversation moves despite what many would initially dismiss as a superficial statement of need.

Preparatory change talk describes the part of the offender that feels positively about change. Yet the offender may still be ambivalent about change, despite the presence of preparatory change talk in continuing dialogue. The second form of change talk—mobilizing change talk—indicates that the person is moving closer to change, and has resolved ambivalence sufficiently to tip the balance in the direction of change. In our example of climbing the hill or mountain, mobilizing change talk moves the offender more rapidly downhill, toward the end goal of behavior change. Three forms of mobilizing change talk signal such movement. These are commitment, activation, and taking steps, or CATS.

Commitment

Commitment language is a clear sign of the person's commitment to change. Rather than hesitant statements like "I should" or "I'd like to," commitment language is characterized by strength or certainty, as in

---

BOX 9.2. JOHN DISCUSSES HIS NEED FOR CHANGE

JOHN: I mean . . . I know it needs to be different. I need to take things more seriously this time.

CASE MANAGER: You've thought about how you'd do things differently.

JOHN: Yeah. This time I need to walk the walk and not just talk the talk.

CASE MANAGER: What does that look like for you?

JOHN: Oh, um . . . I don't really know. I guess it's just what they always say in treatment. (*Laughs.*) I know it means to not just say you're gonna do something but to actually do it. What would that look like for me? (*Pauses, thinking.*) Well, first I would have to be more open-minded in treatment. In the past, I really haven't been all that excited about trying new things, and I haven't been all that honest with the therapist about what's really going on. I kept things pretty close. I need to open up and be real about it.

CASE MANAGER: Sounds like a good first step.

"I will" or "I promise." Unfortunately, in working with offenders, you become accustomed to hearing such promises and feeling jaded when there is a lack of follow-through. Good intentions, and even strong commitment, do not invariably lead to success. And offenders, perhaps even more than others who want change, have often been met with criticism or frustration when they voice preparatory change talk. They may prematurely offer assurances of commitment to decrease the person's annoyance with them in the moment, or to receive positive praise. Imagine, for example, an offender who is talking with his frustrated probation officer—perhaps an officer who has heard the same "I really want to change" speech from this offender before. An arched eyebrow, sigh, or even the probation officer shaking her head might prompt a response of "No, really! This time I'm going to do it! I give you my word." This is commitment language, but do you believe it in the same way you would if it came without prompting? Or if it was your first time hearing it? Or from a nonoffender?

We include this only because it may be difficult for you to see mobilizing commitment language as different from preparatory change talk. After hearing it for some time and experiencing the frustration of disappointment, it becomes easy to discount the difference and underestimate the power of commitment language. Ultimately, however, these forms of speech communicate to us that the offender is ready to stop merely considering alternatives and pursue them in a more meaningful way. Evoking additional mobilizing talk signifies the resolution of ambivalence in favor of change and solidifies pursuit of change-supportive alternatives.

Activation

Like commitment language, activation language lets us know that the client is ready to consider what happens next. Take a look at Table 9.1 for some examples of differences between preparatory change talk and activation language.

Note the important differences. Activation involves an indication of preparedness, willingness, or anticipation that is lacking in preparatory change talk. While preparatory change talk still moves the offender closer to change, it can fall short of a reassuring or satisfying answer (though the goal is not to reassure or satisfy the listener). Even activation language can feel that way, particularly if you are expecting a much stronger and more immediate resolution of ambivalence. But remember, if the person could fully resolve ambivalence, make a plan, and move forward without your help, he or she would have done so already. It seems unfair to expect so much in an initial conversation. Yet that is typically what happens. For example, it is common for a treatment provider working with people who have problems to expect that they will immediately solve those problems upon initiating treatment. However, if the person could so simply stop a habitual behavior, they would have done it without treatment. The purpose of treatment is to gradually learn skills that will help them stop. It is the same with MI. You talk with people about change to help them reach a point where they understand their ambivalence, explore options, make a decision, and develop a plan. Within this sequence, activation language is evidence of making a decision and mobilizing effort for a potential plan.

We will discuss what to do with activation language in greater detail

TABLE 9.1. Activation Language, Contrasted with Preparatory Change Talk

Activation language	Preparatory change talk
"I'm ready to talk about treatment."	"I should go to treatment."
"I'm willing to do what it takes to make things up to my family."	"I need to think about my family."
"I'm prepared to do what the court wants this time."	"I want to do what the judge said."
"I'm going to take things more seriously this time."	"I think I can do what I need to do."

in the next chapter. However, when you encounter activation, a natural instinct is to ask for greater detail. A client who says he or she is ready, willing, and prepared for change provides a natural prompt for you to ask what the client plans to do next.

Taking Steps

This type of mobilizing change talk indicates that the offender has already taken initial first steps toward anticipated change. Some examples include statements like:

> "I started walking home a different way—one that doesn't take me past my dealer's apartment."
> "I called and asked about those jobs from the list you gave me."
> "I set up a special draw on my paycheck to start paying on my restitution."
> "I went by the treatment clinic and asked them about when their groups are."

Each of these suggests that the person is more decided about change, and also that he or she has done something about it. Obviously, one can always say that more is needed. The person who avoids his drug dealer's apartment may not be equipped to consistently face urges for drug use, the person who called about jobs may not get any of them, and the person who asked about treatment groups may not actually go to them. The work of change continues. Even so, taking initial steps is a positive sign in the desired direction.

Interspersed within occurrences of change talk, you will also hear sustain talk. Sustain talk—previously subsumed under resistance (Miller & Rollnick, 1991, 2002)—is talk that supports the status quo. It represents the side of ambivalence that is against change. Sustain talk can exhibit the same aspects of DARN as preparatory change talk. See Table 9.2 for some relevant examples. These statements are easy to imagine coming from any offender. They predict the direction the offender will choose, and we can see the offender moving to the bottom of the hill, only on the side on which he or she began.

Sustain talk can also take the form of mobilizing talk, or CATS. You may hear statements like "I plan to keep dealing drugs; it's a good source of income" (commitment language); "I'm prepared to accept the risks of what I'm doing now" (activation language); or even "I already contacted my friend who has helped me sell stuff in the past to see if

TABLE 9.2. Sustain Talk, Expressed as Desire, Ability, Reason, and Need

Desire
_____

"I love how I feel when I'm using."

"I don't want to stop seeing my friends, even if they do things I'm not supposed to be around."

Ability
_____

"I've gone to treatment over and over, and nothing ever changes."

"I can make better choices without anyone telling me what to do."

"It's not like anything I do makes a difference. Everyone has already made up their minds about me."

Reason
_____

"Getting high is the only thing that helps me feel better after a bad day."

"Going to that group makes me feel even worse—all those people looking at me, judging me."

Need
_____

"I don't need treatment. What I need is a job, and a place to stay where people will get off my back."

"This is just how I am. No amount of treatment or restrictions is gonna change that."

"What I need to do is stop listening to the people who criticize me. They don't know anything about me."

there's a way for me to get some extra cash" (taking steps). Certainly any of these are discouraging in your work with offenders. You might balk at such talk, fighting an immediate urge to challenge it. Immediate confrontation will result in a more firmly entrenched commitment to the status quo. Instead, in our next chapter, we review key strategies for responding to sustain talk. But in the meantime, remember that within sustain talk also lies truth. If there wasn't some benefit to the status quo—despite punitive consequences, or benefits we do not understand—the offender would have already given up problematic behavior. Dismissing sustain talk as "wrong" suggests a greater need for accurate empathy and compassion to get you back on track with MI.

AMBIVALENCE AND DISCREPANCY

Change talk and sustain talk represent the different aspects of the client's ambivalence. Both are valid pieces of how the offender feels about making a change versus keeping things as they are. Preparatory change talk indicates that the balance has tipped a bit in favor of change, at least enough that the client is familiar with desire, ability, reason, and need for change. Mobilizing change talk may indicate preliminary decisions in favor of change. Sustain talk is not resistance to change but instead a normal part of the person that remains conflicted and desires things as they are. Ambivalence, therefore, underlies both.

Here, we consider four forms of ambivalence and how they influence the nature of change and sustain talk in your conversations with the offender:

1. *Approach–approach.* The offender is divided between two positive choices, or a win–win situation. Still, a decision must be made. For our client John, it may mean choosing between first improving his relationship with his wife and finding ways to increase positive mood. Both are things he would like and that would benefit him, but perhaps he can only start with one due to time constraints, limited resources, or other environmental demands. While he may be pleased with selecting either, he may voice postdecisional regret (e.g., "Well, I do feel a lot better day to day, but I still think maybe I should have spent more time working on my marriage."). The challenge for the listener is to catalog change talk in support of one decision as opposed to change talk in support of another option. Sustain talk may emerge when the person feels so frustrated by having to choose that he or she says it would be easier to just avoid a decision altogether and leave things as they are.

2. *Avoidance–avoidance.* This is the classic "between a rock and a hard place" scenario. The client has two or more options, both or all of which are potentially unpleasant. For the client, it appears to be a lose–lose situation. Imagine the client who must give up drugs or alcohol, while still knowing the distress of withdrawal, intensity of cravings, or prospect of incarceration should he or she fail to abstain. Both options (i.e., quitting and not quitting) carry significant negative implications; still, a choice must be made. Similarly, a client may know that treatment is needed but not be able to pay for the cost of treatment, knowing that refusing treatment leads to revocation of probation or other negative sanctions from the court. Here, sustain talk may be more prominent as the client focuses on both the negative aspects of complying with orders and the negative aspects of failing to comply. Preparatory change talk may be more common than mobilizing change talk, since movement toward change only emphasizes the negative factors associated with making a change.

3. *Approach–avoidance.* This scenario involves only one choice, but one that has both positive and negative aspects to it. Our client John, for example, knows that he needs to attend counseling to help with his mood and anger problems. He knows that it would be good for him to feel better. However, he also knows that he will have to talk about things that make him uncomfortable, and that he will have to be open about deeply personal matters that make him feel vulnerable. The client in this situation will likely exhibit both preparatory and mobilizing change talk, interspersed with sustain talk that emphasizes the negative aspects of change rather than glorifying or supporting the status quo.

4. *Double approach–avoidance.* This is perhaps the most difficult dilemma for both offenders and listeners. Much like the approach–avoidance dilemma, there are positive and negative aspects to potential change. However, with the double approach–avoidance scenario, there are two or more options that carry both negative and positive implications. Let us revisit John's ambivalence. He wants to stop using drugs and alcohol, though this has been one of his primary coping strategies for dealing with high levels of stress, anxiety, and depression. He also wants to improve his relationship with his wife and children, though this requires a great deal of effort—securing a job and earning more money to decrease arguments over finances, learning new ways of interacting with others, and also spending time that he fears he does not have. The more he considers his first option—stopping his drug and alcohol abuse—he may be faced with vulnerability and increased emotional distress. If he moves to another option instead, he may improve his relationships and the lives of his wife and children, but he must also work harder than perhaps he feels himself capable of doing, with only the potential (not a promise) of payoff. With this kind of dilemma, you will hear a great deal of both change and sustain talk, often alternating and intensifying as ambivalence remains unresolved.

Discrepancy is also relevant during the process of evoking. As was discussed in Chapter 7, discrepancy is the realization of where you are in relation to where you would like to be. Evoking discrepancy is a good way to facilitate change. Once clients begin to form a clearer picture of where they would like to be, you can expect to hear greater preparatory change talk. However, if the offender is too far away from that desired state, sustain talk that reflects inability or lack of confidence will emerge.

How do you recognize discrepancy during this phase of the conversation? As with focusing, discrepancy can be more fully explored through a discussion of values. No one is truly "unmotivated"; everyone wants *something*. When the offender identifies his or her primary values, it provides an opportunity to compare the current state with a value-based ideal. Values should be intrinsic; offenders are often encouraged to adopt the values of society or those in the criminal justice system rather than exploring their own. They may readily agree with the values of the dominant society, though it is important that you not assume moral superiority when discussing values like following the rules versus independence, or taking care of oneself versus taking care of others, or finding new sources of social support versus loyalty to longtime friends and family. Remember, too, that many offenders have been repeatedly told how far they are from where they need to be, when each person is an individual and may be further from or closer to their goals in any given moment.

At this point, your role is to give the client pause. Questions that you and the client can explore together include:

"Where have you been with . . . [this topic, target, goal, etc.]?"
"Where are you now with that?"
"Where do you want to be?"
"What would it take to get there?"
"How do you see yourself getting to that point?"
"What would help you get there?"

Such open questions get at the heart of discrepancy, evoking preparatory and mobilizing change talk that can move the client forward. Still, sustain talk is present, particularly when the offender feels a lack of confidence or ability to achieve his or her goals.

A reminder is warranted—respecting and acknowledging autonomy is critical as you evoke and explore change talk. Goals, values, and discrepancy all belong to the client. While you may feel some pressure to address your own goals, or those of your agency or the court, pushing a specific agenda without permission or in contrast with the client's agenda will move you further from making meaningful change. Because you are not an intrinsic part of the offender's world, your own goals are secondary to those most valued by the offender. If you find it difficult to explore change talk or address sustain talk in a way that honors autonomy (and it will happen, eventually), revisit the discussions in Chapters 7 and 8 about when goals differ, and perhaps have an open conversation with the client about differences of opinion in a nonjudgmental and non-directive way.

EVOKING WITH OFFENDER POPULATIONS

Evoking is a process requiring self-evaluation on the part of the client. You become a kind of mirror. For any client, this may be a difficult process that provokes feelings of vulnerability. Offenders face unique challenges as they strive to explore what it means to change. First, this is a population from whom sustain talk may be particularly high. This is true for a number of reasons, including past efforts by others to seemingly force or coerce them into change, as well as the perceived or real benefits of maintaining the status quo. The client may become more entrenched in believing, verbalizing, and clinging to sustain talk due to past efforts at challenging it. Because of this, you may find yourself dealing with more sustain talk than you had expected, and the client may even be more committed to sustain talk than he or she expected. Our advice is to simply go with it, acknowledge the reality of the offender's world, and continue to reflect ambivalence.

A second issue evidenced more strongly in working with offenders is that past efforts at change have likely been unsuccessful or unsupported by others in the client's social network. A core component of preparatory change talk is ability, and if clients have failed in previous attempts at change, they may begin to doubt their ability to make similar changes in the future. Hearing things like "I've gone to treatment before, and it didn't do any good" or "Nothing ever really gets better, no matter how hard I try" will likely evoke your own righting reflex—you want to argue against the client to bolster his or her confidence. This, however, will only make the offender argue against his or her ability to make meaningful change, and that is clearly not the goal. Evoking elicits abilities and confidence that lie within, while recognizing that offenders may have quite some way to go.

Also, offenders face realistic deficits that may limit their ability to conceptualize and imagine lasting change. While it is not our intention to focus on these deficits, or to make assumptions about the offender because of them, it is important to remember that many offenders face limited resources, lack of good or prosocial role models, or problems coping with stress and environmental demands in adaptive and healthy ways. Such factors also increase sustain talk and can make evoking a slower and more deliberate process.

What is your role in this? Put simply, it is to guide the offender toward change, and to facilitate hope, strength, and confidence. Find the inherent strength, ability, and desire for meaningful change that lies within. It is there—no matter how challenging the conversation may be. There has to be some inherent spark of desire, ability, reason, or need, or the client would have given up already. The offender is talking to you. That alone is evidence of something that can be elicited, encouraged, and grown into more lasting change.

> *There has to be some inherent spark of desire, ability, reason, or need, or the client would have given up already.*

CHAPTER 10

EVOKING IN PRACTICE

Our dilemma is that we hate change and love it at the same
time; what we really want is for things to remain the same
but get better.
                                        —SYDNEY J. HARRIS

It is one thing to talk about evoking the offender's own reasons for
change but quite another to actually do it. Change talk reflects the side
of the person that wants to change—that side that knows all the reasons
in favor of changing and desires a better life. Sustain talk reflects the
other side of the person—the side that feels fear, self-doubt, and the
desire to keep things as they are. The task for us is to elicit change talk
while still responding to the client's sustain talk in an empathetic and
interested manner. Can you allow for both? And in a way that does not
imply that you are really (maybe not so implicitly) cheering for change?
There is always a need to evoke confidence and hope for the future. But
our goal is not to put pressure on you, or on the client. Evoking is a process, and one that naturally has its own pace.

In this chapter, we devote our attention to the practice of evoking.
In Chapter 9, we spoke to the need for identifying and understanding
change talk and sustain talk, or the two sides of the coin of ambivalence.
We differentiated preparatory change talk from mobilizing change talk,
as well as their counterparts in the realm of sustain talk. We also highlighted important realities of evoking change talk with offenders, all
the more important because offenders may face greater challenges and
setbacks than other clients. Now it is time to move into strategies that
help you evoke change with your offender clients. There are four primary components to this—eliciting change talk, deepening change talk,

140

responding to sustain talk, and instilling hope and building confidence. Each of these is important, and they are interrelated, requiring careful consideration and practice of your new MI skills.

ELICITING CHANGE TALK

Why care so much about change talk? After all, once the client has decided to change, won't he or she just *do it*? While it is true that many people may have a distinct moment of reaching a decision and never going back, this may not be the typical path. Instead, clients often travel a meandering path, so that even though they move forward, there are obstacles, switchbacks, and times when they stop a bit along the road. The goal of evoking is to keep them moving, and to do what you can to ensure that the movement is in a forward direction.

Change talk is the means through which the person stays on the path and keeps moving in a forward direction. Change talk is also the way of gauging the person's inner voice about change. In fact, it is most effective when the change talk is his or her own rather than yours (thus, why you evoke it from within *the client*). By giving voice to change talk, clients talk themselves into change. Sometimes the person's inner voice remains unsure. Consider also that many people say they are ready for change before they are truly ready to begin the work involved. Deepening and reinforcing change talk helps those who need greater resolve before moving forward into action.

One can accomplish this in varying ways, which will be illustrated throughout this section. This is not an exhaustive list of strategies; nor is it a checklist that must be fully completed for you to "do it right" when eliciting change talk from your client. Instead, remain mindful of what your client says in response to what you are doing. If you hear change talk, keep doing what you have been doing. If you hear sustain talk that supports the problem, it may be time to try something different. You will have plenty of opportunity to make adjustments as the conversation progresses.

> *It is most effective when the change talk is his or her own rather than yours.*

Asking Evocative Questions

When you need something, the easiest and most direct way of getting it is to simply ask. It is no different with change talk. To hear change talk, ask for it. Using DARN (see the preparatory change talk described in Chapter 9) may guide you in formulating evocative questions. Consider the examples provided in Table 10.1. These questions are merely examples or guidelines. We encourage you to be creative in developing your own, with the goal being to evoke or facilitate preparatory change talk. Trying to evoke mobilizing change talk too soon may be difficult, and there are other ways of accomplishing that. For now, your goal is to strengthen the offender's awareness of his or her own desire to change, ability, reason, and need for something different.

A note of caution, however—try to avoid language or tone that evokes shame, defensiveness, or discord. Asking open questions is useful unless they are designed to elicit sustain rather than change talk: "Why haven't you gone to treatment already?"; "Do you like how drugs hurt your family?"; "How could you want to keep losing your temper and hurting people like that?" Take a moment and answer each of these in your head as one of your offenders would. The likely response is one that

TABLE 10.1. Asking Evocative Questions with DARN

Desire: Use words like *want, wish, like,* or *hope.*
- "What do you *want* to see that's different in your life?"
- "What do you *wish* could happen in the next year?"
- "How would you *like* for things to change?"
- "Tell me what you *hope* for when you think about your future."

Ability: Use words like *can, able,* or *could.*
- "What *can* you do when you put your mind to it?"
- "How are you *able* to make this time different than before?"
- "Do you have thoughts about how you *could* improve your situation?"

Reason: Use questions that tap into *why* the person wants to change.
- "Why might you want to go to treatment?"
- "What are the good things about stopping your drug use?"
- "What are the best reasons you might make a change in your life?"
- "How could following the court orders help you?"

Need: Use words like *have to, must, need to,* or *important*; emphasize the urgency of change.
- "What do you *have to* do to make things better for yourself?"
- "What is it that you just *must* do right now?"
- "What is the most serious thing you *need to* do?"
- "How *important* is it to you to make this change now?"

prompts shame or anger, and that evokes discord and shuts down any consideration of change. It may also be helpful at times to explore sustain talk—reasons for keeping the problem—to get a better understanding of the situation, or to side with the part of the person that doesn't want to change. This can provide contrast or voice their own arguments, which is something to do carefully and deliberately. Think ahead about what the answers might be, and craft your words so that the questions truly do evoke change talk rather than shame or humiliation, which rarely promote effective change.

Using the Importance Ruler

A key aspect of preparatory change talk is need. How much does the offender feel he or she *needs* to change? This reflects a gut-based instinct of what *must happen*. One strategy for eliciting change talk about need is using the importance ruler (Butler et al., 1999; Miller & Rollnick, 2013). We present a brief illustration of this with our offender, John, in Box 10.1. In this example, John discusses the importance of attending treatment to improve his mood. Note how his case manager uses the importance ruler and thought-out follow-up questions that elicit and strengthen John's change talk surrounding this issue. What if he said it was a zero? It's possible that you might get such a response, indicating that the offender has no ambivalence about the matter. He or she simply doesn't see it as important, or even a problem. In these instances, work toward exploring ambivalence, developing discrepancy, or perhaps refocusing on something that the client does view as important. It may also be useful to consider the case manager's final question, asking how important the issue might be to others in the offender's life, to broaden and continue the discussion without evoking defensiveness, frustration, or hostility.

Querying Extremes

To increase a person's talk about desire, reason, or need for change, you may find it helpful for the client to consider extremes of change versus not changing. Some examples are provided below. The first three are "worst-case scenario" questions for the offender, prompting him or her to think about extreme consequences of maintaining the status quo. The latter three ask the offender to imagine the best outcomes that could occur if he or she were to make important changes.

**BOX 10.1. USING THE IMPORTANCE RULER
TO ELICIT CHANGE TALK FROM JOHN**

CASE MANAGER: John, you've talked a lot about how going to your therapy group might help with your mood. How important is it for you to make some changes that will help improve your mood?

JOHN: Well, I know it's something I need to do.

CASE MANAGER: Okay, right. So on a scale of 0 to 10, with 0 being completely unimportant, and 10 being the most important, how important would you say it is for you to go to treatment to work on your mood?

JOHN: Well, like maybe a 5 or a 6.

CASE MANAGER: Good. That helps. I'm curious though . . . why are you at a 5 or 6, and not a 2 or a 3? Or even a 0?

JOHN: Well, because it's something I know I really need to work on. No one likes feeling bad all the time, or even some of the time. And I see how much it affects everyone around me—my family, my job, and what the judge thinks of how I'm doing. So it's pretty important.

CASE MANAGER: What would it take for you to go from a 5 or a 6 up to some higher number, like an 8 or 9?

JOHN: I think I'd have to have a better handle on some of the other stuff that's going on in my life. Right now, I have a lot to work on. So while feeling better is important to me, for it to be more important, I'd have to feel like my relationship with my wife, how things are going with my kids, my recovery, and other stuff is under better control. But that's still not saying that I don't think it's important to go to treatment and work on my mood. I know that all of it is related anyway.

CASE MANAGER: That's a good way of looking at things. I wonder though . . . if I were to ask your wife how important she would rate it—improving your mood—what number do you think she would give it?

JOHN: (Laughs.) Probably like a 10. She knows I'm really tough to be around when I'm having a bad day. So she'd say it's the most important thing.

CASE MANAGER: Huh. That's pretty interesting. So it's something you two would agree on as being pretty important.

JOHN: Yeah.

"What worries you the most about continuing your drug use?"

"If you were to keep going along as you have, breaking into cars or selling drugs for extra income, what do you think is the worst that could happen?"

"This judge that gave you probation—he sometimes sends people to jail or prison for violations. Even if you don't see that happening

to you, what do you know about going to jail or prison for a long
time? What would that do to a person's life?"

"What would be the best outcome for you, if you were to go to your
treatment group?"

"If you were able to change all of the things we talked about, how
might things be different in your life?"

"What might happen if you were to succeed in making these
changes?"

Looking Back/Looking Forward

Another useful technique to elicit change talk is for the person to reflect
or look back to a time before the problem existed, comparing it with
his or her present reality: "Can you remember a time when you didn't
have any legal problems? What was that like?" Other questions that call
for looking back may be more specific in providing contrast: "What is
different about the person you were as a young adult—before you were
into drugs or in trouble with the law—versus the person you are today?"
Thinking about a time when things were better for the client as he or she
also considers the present may increase the client's desire for change, or
help the client identify reasons for change. A challenge for some offenders is that they may have experienced legal or other troubles for much of
their lives, and it is difficult for them to remember a time when they did
not have problems or involvement with the court. For these individuals,
looking back may be more difficult. While they may be able to envision
a past with fewer troubles, it may not provide the contrast necessary to
elicit preparatory change talk.

Another important strategy, then, is to look forward into a future in
which the problem no longer exists. Thoughtful questions may prompt
the client to imagine a changed future: "Have you thought about how
your world would be different if you were to make this change?"; "Imagine yourself making this change, and then move forward 5 years, or
10—what's that like?"; "If suddenly a miracle occurred and all of your
legal problems were gone, what would you do first?" These call forth the
person's hope for a better future, and if you are able to pair that better
future with making an important change, it will increase the amount
of preparatory change talk you hear from the client. Similarly, you can
combine this with querying extremes to ask the worst-case-scenario
question: "If you do nothing, and you keep going like you have been,
what will your life look like in 5 years, or 10?" This, however, will not

necessarily lead to hope, though it might still accomplish the goal of initiating more change talk.

Exploring Goals and Values

Understanding and incorporating the person's own goals and values into the conversation is a cornerstone of the spirit and style of MI. This stance assumes that the offender is motivated by his or her own values and priorities. Because the client's goals, values, or priorities may not align precisely with the court's goals, or the values of a particular agency or person within that agency, does not mean that he or she cannot change. Tapping into those goals and values can provoke preparatory change talk. To do this, revisit earlier conversations with the offender about important life goals, strongly held values or beliefs, or other priorities that arose during the processes of engaging and focusing. Ask questions that develop discrepancy, highlighting how the status quo may not be in line with the offender's values, or how making a change would help him or her move closer to a desired goal. Some examples: "How might making this change help you feel more independent and in control of your life?"; "If you were to go to therapy, what would your family think?"; "What you're doing now for money makes you feel disgusted with yourself; what might you be able to do to get your self-respect back?" Such questions should be clearly tied to a value or goal that the client has already expressed. Imposing goals on the offender may provoke defensiveness and is unlikely to elicit productive change talk.

RESPONDING TO CHANGE TALK

Once you hear change talk, it may be tempting to sit back and think that your task is finished. After all, the offender gets it and is going to change, right? Well, maybe. The client is voicing reasons for change and may have even begun mobilizing for more lasting change later, but you still play an important role in continuing the conversation. Change doesn't occur simply through talking about why it's a good idea; how you respond to the offender's change talk will help them stay on the side of change and make a clear decision about what they will do. This occurs, in part, by having the offender compare his or her values with current behavior, as well as examining the offender's own change talk.

The core OARS skills described in Chapter 6 are used in a motivational interview for not only engaging the offender but also for responding to their change talk. Open questions, affirmations, reflections, and summaries provide a careful balance of responding that pulls forth more change talk, facilitates clients talking themselves into change, and causes them to think critically about important next steps for change to occur.

Open Questions

When offenders voice reasons for change, you may have a moment of thinking, "Well, yes . . . that's what everyone's been trying to tell you." Thinking this to yourself diminishes your curiosity about what the client is saying. To respond to change talk in a genuine and helpful manner, remain curious. Curiosity and interest are best conveyed through open questions that elicit greater dialogue and cause the person to think about what he or she has just said. For example, see three differing options for open questions one could use in response to John's statement below:

JOHN: I don't like how I am when I feel angry and can't control it.

CASE MANAGER: What is it that you're like when you're angry? How have you tried to control it before? How will you do something differently the next time you're angry?

The case manager's first question elicits further preparatory change talk that emphasizes reason or need for change. The second question might prompt preparatory change talk focusing on ability, or even mobilizing change talk describing taking steps to change. The third question hones in on commitment language. Each of these questions is designed to bring forth further change talk, depending on the outcome that might be most beneficial to further the conversation.

Affirmations

During the process of engaging, affirmations helped build a positive relationship between you and your offender client. Now, affirmations are a way to recognize and express the value of the client's change talk. Offering positive or encouraging comments can go a long way toward reinforcing the importance of change and instilling confidence in the offender. Some examples of affirmations include: "Good for you!"; "That was really hard work!"; "This is something you really care about."; "I bet others have really noticed how seriously you're taking this."

Reflections

Reflective listening is a skill that permeates the process of MI. As with affirmations, the use of reflections in the initial stages of MI was meant to build rapport and to more fully understand the offender's world. Reflective listening also demonstrated a sense of compassion for the offender's experiences. In evoking, reflection is used very purposefully and thoughtfully to highlight and increase change talk. Simple reflections are useful for checking in and for emphasizing certain statements in support of change, whereas complex reflections can take the conversation deeper and can also make a guess at what change talk has not yet overtly stated. This idea of using a complex reflection to continue the paragraph lets you guess at what would come next, and add in some change talk that seems simmering just beneath the surface. When you reflect change talk, you tend to get more of it. Be careful, though, not to reflect too much sustain talk, or the conversation may become mired in arguments against change rather than for it.

Summaries

During the process of evoking, the purpose of the summary is to collect a bouquet of change talk to present to the offender. The goals of the summary are varied. First, bringing together the elements of change talk that were spread throughout the conversation underscores both preparatory and mobilizing statements. Second, it may strengthen commitment to change. Third, continuing to engage the offender and demonstrate your understanding of his or her dilemma shows that you understand the person's emotions, needs, thoughts, and the very ambivalence that has brought him or her to you. Finally, bringing forth their strongest arguments for change and then prompting them with an open question (the key question) will transition them to planning, the next phase of MI. Different types of summaries may emphasize different goals, and it is likely that you will offer multiple summaries during this phase of the conversation. While earlier use of summaries had a more balanced consideration of the pros and cons of change, or the pros and cons of the status quo, the difference here is that you focus mainly on change talk.

In practice, your use of OARS will contain primarily open questions and reflections, with occasional affirmations and a few selected summaries. The goal of using OARS in evoking is to continually elicit change talk. Each of your questions or statements is intended to bring forth more talk in support of change. Let's consider another conversation with John, as presented in Box 10.2. This is a fairly short exchange, though one in which the case manager is able to offer several complex reflections and keep the conversation moving toward further change talk. The summary emphasizes various aspects of change talk that John has mentioned in this and previous exchanges, and we can imagine that John's response to such a summary would be more preparatory change talk, and maybe even mobilizing change talk that further solidifies his growing commitment to change.

RESPONDING TO SUSTAIN TALK

Conversations may not always go so smoothly. In fact, it is quite common for sustain talk to emerge. This simply reflects the opposite side of the same coin that depicts change talk. Sustain talk is the offender's way of voicing his or her ambivalence, or fears and hesitations in considering important changes. Initial discussions of MI (e.g., Miller & Rollnick,

---

BOX 10.2. USING OARS TO RESPOND TO JOHN'S CHANGE TALK, IN BRIEF

JOHN: I know it's important to get my anger and my moods under control. I might even have to think about taking medication again.

CASE MANAGER: How do you feel about that? [open question]

JOHN: Well, I don't like it. I don't like having to take a pill to make me feel better. I feel like a failure doing that. And I'm trying to get off of the drugs anyway, so it feels like I'm doing something wrong.

CASE MANAGER: You're working so hard. [affirmation] It feels like a step backward, even though you know it will help. [complex reflection]

JOHN: I guess so. Yeah, I know what you mean. I want help though. I don't want to mess up again this time. I just need to get over it, I guess, and get on with treatment.

CASE MANAGER: You're ready. [complex reflection] Here's where we're at. You have a long history of problems with your mood—both depression and anxiety—and because of that you have also had some problems with controlling you anger. It just becomes too much for you. You really want to feel better . . . to feel more stable. You don't like how you feel, or how you are to others, when your moods are out of control. You don't like to feel out of control. You really want things to be different this time. You know that medication is available, and that it might help. You fear of taking medication is real, and at the same time, you know it can help. You want help. You want to give treatment a chance to work this time. What else? [summary]

1991, 2002) conceptualized such talk as resistance, positing that it reflected the client's active resistance to change. However, over time, this view has evolved. The term "resistance" implies a process in which the client is simply trying to be difficult. No one likes it when a person is trying to be difficult—you resent it, and your immediate response is to confront, challenge, or ignore the resistance and keep going. None of these responses is consistent with the spirit of MI.

But here is an important question: Is it really that the person is *trying* to be difficult? What would be the motivation? Making you frustrated and confrontational only serves to make the conversation go worse, and both of you end up feeling bad. Labeling this as an intentional attempt to thwart your best efforts to evoke change talk is pathologizing something that is a normal part of ambivalence. This is why instead it is called "sustain talk," reflecting that it is the other side of ambivalence and not something inherently indicative of hostility, discord, or sabotage.

To be fair, there are times when the conversation with an offender is characterized by hostility and opposition. Offenders are often resentful or angry about their sanctions, or because they are "forced" to talk to someone about their conditions of supervision, treatment needs, or the like. They may have a bad relationship with you for reasons known or unknown, certainly complicating matters. We discuss this further in Chapter 13, though reliance on the spirit of MI and an empathic, collaborative relationship can certainly offset some of the tension. But for the most part, be cautious about interpreting sustain talk as anything other than one side of ambivalence. Here's where MI has most helped to inform correctional work, for example. For decades, if an offender voiced sustain talk and reasons for holding on to problem behavior, correctional officers and therapists viewed this as a form of resistance—an active effort to avoid and fight against change. Not so. Rather, it's natural for an offender to voice both sides of ambivalence, though classifying it as resistance and treating it as such

> *It's natural for an offender to voice both sides of ambivalence.*

gets you nowhere. Worse yet, it prevents you from effectively evoking change talk, damages the relationship, and decreases your own motivation to continue working toward change with the offender.

There are two primary means of responding to sustain talk that will put you and your offender client back on the task of evoking change talk. One of these is reflective responses that use varying forms of reflective statements, and the other is strategic responses, when one must do something beyond just reflecting in a meaningful way. We will now consider each of these in turn, using a number of examples to illustrate these approaches.

Reflective Responses

In Chapters 3 and 6 we described what has been termed *straight reflection*—or the use of simple and complex reflections to revisit what the person has already said. Using straight reflections, you are on alert for the offender's own instances of change talk and use these to reflect more change talk. It is the same for sustain talk, only that you're listening for simple and complex reflections in a way that allow the person to hear and evaluate the validity of his or her own sustain talk. Below is a hypothetical example from a drug and alcohol treatment intake.

> OFFENDER: I don't need treatment. I can stop doing drugs whenever I want to, and without the court being involved.
>
> TREATMENT PROVIDER: You can do it yourself.
>
> OFFENDER: Well, I don't know about that. I probably still would need some help.

Note how upon reflection, the offender realizes that what he or she has said is not completely true—help may be needed. And this realization could decrease commitment to sustain talk and instead lead the offender toward a consideration of the benefits of treatment.

Another type of reflective response is an *amplified reflection*. With this type of statement, you still reflect what the client has said, only you amplify or intensify his or her statement. The contrast may invite the client to think differently about it, prompting him or her to begin defending a need for change. Here, we have several examples that amplify different parts of the offender's sustain talk, leading to preparatory change talk that is far more productive for the conversation.

Example 1

> OFFENDER: This whole thing is ridiculous. The judge really overreacted.
>
> PROBATION OFFICER: You didn't do anything wrong.
>
> OFFENDER: Well, not exactly. I mean, I did break the law. I know I shouldn't have done that. I told myself I wouldn't be like that again. But here I am.

Example 2

OFFENDER: I don't really have a problem with sex offending.

CASE MANAGER: It doesn't bother you at all.

OFFENDER: No, wait! That's not what I meant! I mean, it's wrong and all. And it does bother me. I don't want people to view me as someone with a problem like that. I just really want to feel more in control of it.

Example 3

OFFENDER: My kids need to stop telling people these things.

INTERVIEWER: Because it's none of their business what goes on in the home.

OFFENDER: Yeah, but I guess they live there, too. And when I was a kid I hated to hear my parents fight. Always made me scared. I'm sure they're just scared too, and I don't want that.

The third option is the *double-sided reflection,* a form of reflection that acknowledges both sustain talk and change talk. This kind of statement reflects the competing sides of ambivalence, which is something you may have already incorporated into a summary for the offender. There is an art, however, to using the double-sided reflection. First, be careful about the use of *but* versus *and.* The word *but* tends to negate whatever precedes it. Imagine a performance evaluation in which your supervisor says, "You're a very good employee, *but* . . . . " The only part you will hear is what follows *but.* It serves to negate the fact that your supervisor said you are a good employee. This is simply human nature. Thus, when doing a double-sided reflection, note the difference as depicted in Table 10.2.

Here, we also present examples using *but,* though change talk still follows. It still may be preferable to use *and* so as to diminish the presentation of arguing one side over the other yourself. The decision rests with you, though the emotional valence of the conversation is important. A client who seems to be teetering on the edge of giving more change talk may merit the latter, whereas a client who seems suspicious or hostile may warrant the more balanced approach. If it doesn't work that time, you have plenty of additional opportunities to continue the conversation and get it back on track. The goal is to evoke change talk rather than continuously reflect more sustain talk, as this will detract from the goal of meaningful change.

TABLE 10.2. Double-Sided Reflections: Using the Words *But* versus *And*

Evoking more sustain talk	Evoking change talk
"You want to feel better, *but* it seems like too much work right now."	"It will take a lot of work, *but* you want to feel better."
"Treatment will help, *but* it means that you'll have to talk about your problems in front of people you don't know."	"You may make yourself vulnerable, *and* treatment will help when you do that."
"You know there's a reason for it, *but* your court orders seem unfair."	"Your court orders seem unfair, *but* you know that they're there for a reason."
"You know that your behavior is what gets you out of here sooner, *but* it's so hard to follow rules that feel petty and arbitrary."	"It feels like the rules are petty or arbitrary, *and* still, they may get you out sooner."

Strategic Responses

Though reflective statements can go a long way toward keeping the conversation moving, respectfully giving time to sustain talk while still evoking change talk, and avoiding the righting reflex or the expert trap, they may not always be enough. Here we review five alternative options for responding to sustain talk in a way consistent with evoking and MI as a whole.

Emphasizing Autonomy

Decisions about change always rest with the client. But when you hear a great deal of sustain talk, it may mean that the client has forgotten this, or does not feel in control of the decision during the conversation. Statements from the client like "I can't," "I don't want to," or "I don't need to" are not only sustain talk but also indicate that the client feels a need to assert his or her own independence and autonomy. The client is arguing against change, and it may be because the offender feels pressure—either implicitly or explicitly—from you or others to make a change he or she is not yet committed to. Think of very small children and how they assert their autonomy and independence. By saying *no*. Adults are likely to do the same, though it can manifest itself in the form of sustain talk. Thus, a response that can decrease sustain talk and potentially evoke change talk is to emphasize autonomy in a genuine and serious way.

> "The decision is really up to you."
> "No one can make you do anything you don't want to do. You get
>   to decide."
> "You always have a choice."
> "You can certainly make decisions without being told what to do."

Reframing

When the client gives you sustain talk, there is perhaps more than one way to interpret it. Giving new meaning or perspective to the client's view can shift his or her own view of it as well. See the examples below.

Example 1

OFFENDER: My mom says that if I get sent to jail again, she doesn't want anything to do with me anymore. But maybe that's just who I am, and she'll need to deal with it.

CASE MANAGER: She really cares about you and is scared. It's difficult for her to see you suffering in jail.

Example 2

OFFENDER: I've been in here so long, it's not like I'm ever really going to get out.

CORRECTIONAL OFFICER: You have a lot of time to figure out what you really want!

In these examples, the listener invites the offender to see the situation in a different way. The first offender's mother isn't trying to deny him who he is—she is merely worried about him. The second offender's frustration over a lengthy incarceration can be viewed instead as ample opportunity to reflect and make a reasoned decision. The goal is not for the offender to agree with the listener or to negate the sustain talk. That would invite confrontation. Instead, the goal is to provide a slight shift in tone that may facilitate movement forward with evoking.

Agreeing, with a Twist

This strategy is a combination of good reflection and reframing. A good reframe is sometimes made stronger or more striking with a reflective statement preceding it. Delivering it without sarcasm or in a way that suggests you're trying to make a particular point is a vital skill. Some examples are highlighted below.

- (*The offender has just noted that all of his friends are criminals, and going to treatment and making changes would cost him his friendships.*) "Your friends are a part of your life. It's worth keeping them, even if you have to go back to prison to do it."
- (*The offender has just described how following the rules never seems to work.*) "You try and try, and it's so frustrating. You're an amazingly persistent person!"
- (*The offender says that the treatment group she was assigned to has people in it she doesn't like, and that it won't be all that helpful to her.*) "It's hard to talk about such personal things in front of people you don't like. I wonder, though, if you might find ways of being an example of treatment success to those people."

It's a very delicate process. Reframing is highly individualized and also specific to your relationship with any given offender. Some people might respond in a desired direction, while it's possible that others may perceive it as sarcasm or playing games. If in doubt, use another approach. But this can be a powerful way to prompt self-reflection and preparatory change talk.

Running Head Start

Sometimes the client gives you very little change talk to work with, or the balance is so strongly tipped in the direction of maintaining the status quo that it seems impossible to get a foothold on evoking change talk. Yet you don't want to get into an argument with the client. Assume that the sustain talk, however, has an opposite. With a running head start, you directly ask about the other side of the offender's ambivalence. See the exchange below between a correctional officer and an offender who has been referred for anger management.

> OFFENDER: I don't have an anger problem. I just don't get why people can't see that.
>
> CORRECTIONAL OFFICER: You're frustrated.
>
> OFFENDER: Yeah! Just frustrated, but not angry. There's a difference.
>
> CORRECTIONAL OFFICER: Treatment makes it seem like there's a problem.

OFFENDER: Right, and there's no problem! People make such a big deal out of nothing.

CORRECTIONAL OFFICER: Why do you think the medical unit made the referral?

OFFENDER: Well, my blood pressure's too high. I mean, there are meds for that, right? It's not because I'm always angry. But I did get angry . . . no, frustrated . . . with the doctor when he said that I should think about anger management, too. Like I have problems. I work hard to control myself.

CORRECTIONAL OFFICER: You don't like that you were referred for treatment. Have you heard anything about treatment that might make it helpful to you?

OFFENDER: Well, I don't know. Some of the other guys say that the therapist is pretty good. That she really listens.

CORRECTIONAL OFFICER: Okay. That helps to know. What else?

OFFENDER: It might get the doctor off my back. Who knows? Maybe it would help my blood pressure. And it could be good to feel less tense.

The correctional officer explicitly asks if there might be anything helpful about treatment. As is true with agreeing with a twist, it relies on your relationship with the client. If you know asking such a question might trigger hostility or damage the relationship, use a different strategy. But sometimes it takes very little to prompt the other side of ambivalence that simmers beneath.

Coming Alongside

Where can you and the offender agree, facilitating greater engagement? There are many possibilities for this, especially when you use accurate empathy: *feeling bad after coming from a court hearing, having someone tell you what to do, or difficulty making appointments and keeping up with responsibilities.* Coming alongside can also be used in other situations. Sometimes, it seems there is nothing else to do to break through sustain talk. It's not necessarily because the person is hostile, angry, or "resistant," but because nothing else has worked. Or in some cases, you find that the person makes a really good case for the status quo. This isn't a signal to give up. But something that may still work is coming alongside, or joining with the offender to reestablish accurate empathy and move the conversation forward: "It sounds like it's just too much right now"; "You have so many stressors, and the idea of dealing with one more is simply too much"; "How could you possibly do more than you have already?"; "Blood from a turnip"; "Maybe you should just stick with what's working for now." It's very possible that such a response may generate some preliminary change talk, or at the worst, strengthen your relationship with the offender and keep him or her engaged.

EVOKING HOPE AND CONFIDENCE

Offenders are plagued by a lack of hope for the future. Lengthy sentences, court restrictions, and limited educational, financial, and community resources reinforce their belief that a better life may not be possible. When hope is in short supply, we mistakenly think that they prefer a life of risk, fear, and disappointment.

The same is true for confidence. Many offenders lack confidence in themselves as well as their own abilities to make positive changes. Previous failures, criticism from others, and stigma damage their fragile sense of self-efficacy. How can they possibly trust themselves to make things better when they haven't been able to thus far?

Hope and confidence are deeply personal. Hope is the idea that things can improve. That something will happen. That effort will be worth it. Confidence adds to this—not only does the offender believe that things can be better, but that he or she can make it happen. That change is intentional. That they can impact the outcome. MI is intended to build the offender's hope and confidence so that change is intrinsic and lasting. This begins with the spirit of MI and extends throughout, evoking what comes from within each offender client.

Evoking Hope

A first step is instilling hope. Hope is something that crosses lines of culture, gender, socioeconomic status, age, and other demographic divides. Religious or spiritual traditions, existential considerations of human nature, and scientific views of motivation and perseverance all include elements of hope. It's simply what keeps us going. Hope is an important consideration, as it is a significant predictor of successful change (e.g., Snyder, 1994). One goal of MI is to keep the client in the conversation, with the assumption that change talk and exploring ambivalence and discrepancy will activate the client's hope.

Unlike confidence, which will be discussed in a moment, hope is something inherent within. As much as we, as helpers, would love to "give" offenders hope, it is not a quality or characteristic that we can simply implant and let grow. Nor is it something we can cheerlead or install. In some cases, hope can be nurtured by external situations, but more often "feeling hopeful" is something internal, or something to be evoked and summoned from within. Find what hope exists, and nurture it. One method of doing this is affirmation. For example: "You must really care about this; you've put so much work into your treatment this time!" Or: "You put in so many job applications this time. One of them is bound to be the right one for you." Affirming positive steps and the offender's indications of hope will in turn increase hope. Similarly, reflection can be used to emphasize hope in the offender's story. Find elements of hope and reflect them back, or use a summary of reflective statements to propel the conversation forward.

It's easy to think that the person has no hope. Offenders have challenging and complicated lives, and they often come to treatment at the behest of others. Still, they have a choice. They don't have to talk to you. The fact that they are willing to stay engaged in the conversation implies some degree of hope. Otherwise, they would spend their time on something else, abandoning the process entirely.

Building Confidence

A second step is building confidence. There is an interactive relationship between hope and confidence—a change in one effects a change in the other. Building confidence leads to an increase in hope. Both are needed for change to occur. Here, we discuss a number of strategies for building confidence in your offender client.

Confidence Talk

Like change talk or sustain talk, confidence talk is a specific type of client speech that communicates the speaker's position. It indicates the speaker's confidence in his or her ability to make needed changes. Preparatory change talk focusing on ability will often mirror confidence talk. Ask open questions to elicit confidence talk, including questions like these: "How might you go about doing this?"; "What will help you make this change?"; "What is a good first step you can take?" Use reflective statements and affirmations to highlight and evoke further confidence talk from the offender. See a brief example below.

OFFENDER: It just seems like a lot to do at once.

PAROLE OFFICER: Where might you start? [open question]

OFFENDER: Well, I guess I could think about finding some new friends. You know, hanging around with people who aren't always getting in trouble themselves.

PAROLE OFFICER: You've thought about this. [affirmation] How might you go about doing that? [open question]

OFFENDER: Well, my mom really wants me to start going to church with her. It means a lot to her. And I guess I could meet some different people there.

PAROLE OFFICER: People who are not like the ones you usually hang out with. [reflection] And it would make your mom happy. [reflection]

OFFENDER: Yeah, and it's not like it's hard. I can go with her any Sunday. She knows a lot of people there because she's gone there for years. So it's not like I'd have to be by myself.

PAROLE OFFICER: She could introduce you to people. [reflection]

OFFENDER: I can do that. It's a start.

In this brief exchange, the parole officer has not only elicited mobilizing change talk, but has also increased the offender's confidence about taking an early step toward building new relationships that may be more prosocial and supportive of change. Words reflective of ability, like *could* and *can,* suggest growing confidence.

Confidence Ruler

Earlier in this chapter we discussed the importance ruler. In the same way, we can use the confidence ruler to strengthen the offender's confidence in his or her ability to make a change. Asking, "How confident are you that you could change if you decided to? On a scale of 0 to 10, with 0 being not at all confident, and 10 the most sure you've ever been, where are you now?" is a way to evaluate confidence. Follow-up questions similar to those with the importance ruler, like "Why are you at a 5 and not a 3?" or "What would it take to go from a 3 to a 7?" can help further the conversation.

Giving Information and Advice

As we noted in the latter section of Chapter 6, there are times when it may be appropriate to give information or advice and still stay within the spirit of MI. Offenders may lack confidence in their ability to change because they don't have the facts. In these instances, information or advice, offered as part of a menu of options, may help strengthen confidence. Note that this wouldn't be telling them something that they already know, but instead helping them navigate an area that remains murky or unclear. For example, a person recently released from a lengthy incarceration may ask, "What kind of job could I get with no college degree and a felony conviction?" A response might be to talk about jobs available in the community, job training opportunities, or a range of options chosen by other offenders in similar circumstances.

Identifying and Affirming Strengths

Offenders are used to hearing everything that they've done wrong, or what their deficits or problems are. MI offers us the opportunity to be more strengths-focused in our work. Affirming the offender's strengths increases confidence and links useful skills and abilities with the potential for change. We refer the reader to the list of attributes in Figure 10.1, which you can discuss with your client using open questions, affirmations, and reflective statements. This exercise can elicit not only confidence talk but change talk as well.

Reviewing Past Successes

No matter how difficult the past, everyone has had some success with change. Small indicators of success, as well as the major ones, are worthy of your attention. While it might be tempting to focus on the time the person quit smoking for a full year, also bring up the times when he or she quit for a few days, or a week at a time. Each of those instances can give you rich information about change processes for that individual. It will also remind the client of the number of times success has been possible.

What's important here is to get detailed information about the person's previous success. Not just that it happened, but how, what got in the way, what helped, and how he or she made the decision to finally do it. All of these will help the client better understand him- or herself and will help set the stage for other changes you have been discussing. Knowing, for example, that a past success on probation involved family support, job stability, coping with stressors ahead of time, and avoiding negative attitudes can map onto a current period of probation for that client, even if the circumstances are different.

Accepting	Committed	Flexible	Persevering	Stubborn
Active	Competent	Focused	Persistent	Thankful
Adaptable	Concerned	Forgiving	Positive	Thorough
Adventuresome	Confident	Forward-looking	Powerful	Thoughtful
Affectionate	Considerate	Free	Prayerful	Tough
Affirmative	Courageous	Happy	Quick	Trusting
Alert	Creative	Healthy	Reasonable	Trustworthy
Alive	Decisive	Hopeful	Receptive	Truthful
Ambitious	Dedicated	Imaginative	Relaxed	Understanding
Anchored	Determined	Ingenious	Reliable	Unique
Assertive	Die-hard	Intelligent	Resourceful	Unstoppable
Assured	Diligent	Knowledgeable	Responsible	Vigorous
Attentive	Doer	Loving	Sensible	Visionary
Bold	Eager	Mature	Skillful	Whole
Brave	Earnest	Open	Solid	Willing
Bright	Effective	Optimistic	Spiritual	Winning
Capable	Energetic	Orderly	Stable	Wise
Careful	Experienced	Organized	Steady	Worthy
Cheerful	Faithful	Patient	Straight	Zealous
Clever	Fearless	Perceptive	Strong	Zestful

FIGURE 10.1. Some characteristics of successful changers. From Miller (2004).

Brainstorming

A familiar problem-solving technique is to brainstorm, or think of as many solutions or ideas as possible to choose from. This is the strategy that offers the most choice and facilitates autonomy while also building confidence. Some ideas will seem relevant but out of reach, while others will be both relevant and achievable. Encourage clients to be creative as they consider all the possibilities before them. This also evokes their hope that the future can be better, or at the least, different from their current reality, where the problem still exists.

Reframing

Earlier in this chapter we introduced the idea of reframing, a common technique for looking at an issue from another perspective. Offenders may lack confidence in their ability to change due to past efforts that have not met their expectations. In other words, they have tried and failed. But rather than viewing these as failed attempts, reframing them as a sign of hope that clients have kept trying, or that each attempt brings them closer to the final goal, may inspire confidence in their ability to try another time.

In the same way, offenders may see many obstacles in their way as they contemplate change. Unsupportive family members, limited resources, low frustration tolerance, or restricted options may negatively impact an offender's confidence. Reframing these obstacles as "challenges" to be overcome, or as signs that the person can use his or her strengths creatively, can deter such perceived challenges from damaging confidence.

Hypothetical Thinking

Sometimes we are better able to think about a situation when it seems distant, or when it is happening to someone else rather than ourselves. Such a change in perspective can also increase our confidence that change is possible. Ask a person, "Can you do this?" and they may likely say no. Ask them, "Could someone else do this?" and they have greater confidence. See an example below.

> OFFENDER: I just don't know how I would do it.
>
> CORRECTIONAL OFFICER: Seems out of reach for you. Imagine you were someone else. How might they go about it?

Alternatively, you could ask the person to imagine him- or herself in the future, looking back after a change had already been made.

> CORRECTIONAL OFFICER: What if it's 5 years from now, and you've been granted parole and time out your sentence. What do you think you would have done to get there?
>
> OFFENDER: Well, probably gotten a job. And stayed away from the drugs.
>
> CORRECTIONAL OFFICER: You were able to do that.
>
> OFFENDER: Yeah. I would have gone to treatment and taken it seriously this time. And probably been honest with my family about what was going on. They would have helped me.
>
> CORRECTIONAL OFFICER: How might you do some of those things?
>
> OFFENDER: I can look into getting back into the substance abuse

classes. I dropped out before. I can always go back, they said. Doesn't hurt to start that before getting out.

All of these are ways to elicit hope and build confidence, leading to more change talk and stronger commitment to lasting change. But this is not the last stop in the MI process. In the next chapter we introduce planning, a process that helps you turn engaging, focusing, and evoking into a workable plan to make committed change a reality for your offender clients.

CHAPTER 11

DEVELOPING A PLAN

No one was ever lost on a straight road.
—INDIAN PROVERB

If MI is a journey, planning is examining the map to determine how to reach your chosen destination. You have a relationship between the traveler and helpful guide (engaging), a map of possible destinations (focusing), and the dedication, momentum, and talent to survive the trip (evoking). But how will you get there? For offenders, the route may not be straight or easy. *You need a plan.*

The plan is the part you may most enjoy. Planning feels easy in comparison to the challenge of building rapport with a person who is justifiably suspicious of the process, navigating the back-and-forth dynamics of ambivalence, and searching for change talk amidst hopelessness and fear of the unknown. Developing the plan, however, is not always easy. It is tempting to rush ahead too quickly, overlooking obstacles and making wrong turns along the way. You may also face the temptation to surrender your role as a guide for that of driver, dictating where the client should go and how best to get there.

In this chapter, we will review signs of readiness for planning and important goals of planning, as well as who is involved in developing a plan with offenders. Similarly, we will discuss commitment—a key factor that links motivation to sustained efforts at change. This includes important strategies for consolidating commitment into a plan, maintaining commitment throughout the change process, sustainable planning, and reinforcing gradual signs of progress toward change.

164

FROM CHANGE TALK TO PLAN

How does evoking change talk lead to planning? The plan is an extension of change talk, making things more specific. Within change talk lies what is needed to move forward. The client has given you desire, reason, ability, and/or need for change (i.e., DARN; see Chapter 9). He or she may have also provided commitment language, activating language, and maybe even early approximations of larger changes (i.e., CATS; see Chapter 9) with the movement from evoking to planning. Each of these tells us something about needed specificity. Planning calls for a guiding style, as has been true of other processes in MI. As the listener, you have what you need to reflect back change talk that will coalesce into a collaborative plan for change.

Developing this collaborative plan involves both planning for discrete, specific behavioral changes (short-term) and planning for broader, overarching commitments (long-term). Including elements of both into the plan will facilitate success. There are also systemic commitments—offenders are part of a larger criminal justice system that tells them how to make these changes. To them, the system is demanding and impatient. There are understandably elements of the plan that offenders would not have selected for themselves, though they may still understand the necessity for change. For example, an offender client in need of treatment for substance-related concerns may readily agree that therapy will help him or her in that effort, though the client may prefer another treatment provider over the one who is contracted with the probation office.

Importantly, there are multiple players involved in developing an offender's change plan. The court or other agencies, individuals within those systems, and outside treatment or service providers all play a role. The court or a parole board, for example, dictates conditions that must be met. A parole office has its standard practices. Individual parole officers have mechanisms for assisting offenders in meeting their requirements. And treatment providers develop a treatment plan with each client. Your role in this process may even differ from these. So there are not only multiple commitments, but potentially multiple plans. The process of planning in MI is meant to bring these together into something navigable for the offender.

CONSOLIDATING COMMITMENT INTO A PLAN

When is a person ready? When do we know it is time to move on— from building motivation for change to starting the planning process and consolidating growing commitment to change? Once again consider behavior change as a trek up a steep hill. At some point you reach the summit and start down the other side. It is at this point that mobilizing change talk occurs, and the transition to planning becomes more evident. But how do you know when your offender client has reached the hilltop? This is one of the least-studied conditions in the behavior change process—when someone is *about* ready to change (Prochaska, DeClimente, & Norcross, 1992a). It's easy to spot reluctance, just as it is also obvious when clients engage in actual change efforts. More subtle is when an offender client is ready to turn the corner. Signals and signs of being "almost there" are less well known. Miller and Rollnick (2002) note seven signs of readiness to change:

1. *Decreased resistance.* The client stops arguing, interrupting, denying, or objecting.
2. *Decreased questions about the problem.* The client seems to have sufficient information about his or her problem to stop asking as many questions. There is a sense of reaching the finish.
3. *Resolve.* The client appears to have reached a resolution, and thus may appear more peaceful, relaxed, calm, unburdened, or settled. Sometimes this occurs following a period of anguish, anger, or tearfulness.
4. *Engagement in change talk.* The client offers change talk (see Chapters 9 and 10), speaking about intention to change ("I need to do something"), concern ("This worries me"), optimism ("I can beat this") or recognition of the problem ("I guess this has turned serious").
5. *Increased questions about change.* The client asks what he or she could do about the problem and how people do go about change when the decide they time is right.
6. *Envisioning.* The client begins to talk about how life might be after a change, to anticipate difficulties if a change is made, or to discuss advantages of change. Offender clients look ahead and often find obstacles. They may make statements such as "But how I get the babysitter to come that early so I can attend the program?" Or "I'm not sure I'll be able to catch the bus at that time." Envisioning may be incorrectly interpreted as sustain talk. If we don't become sensitive to envisioning and stay open and aware to when the client "is close," we may lose the opportunity to move ahead.
7. *Experimenting.* If the client has had time between conversations,

he or she may have begun experimenting with possible change approaches (e.g., going to an Alcoholics Anonymous meeting without being told to, going without drinking for a few days, reading a self-help book).

What then? When you notice one or more of these signs in your client, it would seem this is the time to find out if you're close to the summit of the hill. Remember, however, that testing to see if your offender client is ready does not involve pushing them and hoping for the best. Sometimes it is best to simply ask: "What do you think about how you might go about it?"; "Are you willing to start moving into how you might develop a plan, or is it too soon for that?" For some clients, the directness of such questions is refreshing and moves you forward. However, for others, lingering sustain talk bars the way. Thus, there are also strategies to lead into it more gently, maintaining your collaborative partnership and a focus on the client's own words. One way of doing this is recapitulation, or a summary of change talk, followed by a key question and a deliberate pause. Recapitulation involves taking note of the client's change talk (i.e., DARN CATS) and reflecting it back to him or her in a way that accurately summarizes the main impetus for change. Here, sustain talk need not be completely ignored, though it should usually be minimized. A double-sided reflection can fit well; you begin with a prominent argument against change and follow that with the client's own statements in support of change.

This is one of the least-studied conditions in the behavior change process—when someone is about ready to change.

Next, the key question is an open-ended question that prompts the client to think about what comes next. Some examples of these are provided below (Miller & Rollnick, 2013, p. 265):

"So what do you think you'll do?"
"Where does all of this leave you?"
"So what's next?"
"I wonder what you might do."

The key question focuses on the client's autonomy. Asking broadly about a plan is not the same as asking for commitment, or even soliciting specific action items. Instead, a summary serves as a review of change talk that sits with the offender for a moment, while the key question allows him or her to think about next steps without becoming directive or prescriptive. Following this, a deliberate pause from you allows the client room to think. Your silence communicates your interest and the value of the client's input.

Let us examine what this might look like with our offender client John, whom you have met in previous chapters. John's case manager reflects a bit of John's sustain talk, noting fears that he can't handle all that is being asked of him, following it with a skillful summary of John's change talk and the key question.

> "John, you have a lot riding on you at the moment. It's a lot of pressure, and it seems like people expect too much. At the same time, you know that you can't go on like you have been. Something needs to change. You want a better relationship with your wife—your family. You want better things for your children. You want them to look at their dad and be proud of what you have accomplished. You want your wife to feel like she can count on you. And you want to feel better! You are tired of going back and forth between being angry and sad, and you need something that will help you cope that doesn't leave you in the place that alcohol and drugs do. You know you can do treatment—you've done it before. And you've started looking for a job that will help you pay for your treatment and your family's needs. There's a part of you that knows things will get better. You just feel that part inside of you. *So what do you think you will do?*"

This summary brings forth John's own preparatory and mobilizing change talk, as well as his sense of hope and confidence. The key question doesn't push for any specific answer, or even a deliberate commitment. It is an open, rather than closed, question. How John answers lets you know if you need to back up, continuing to evoke motivation for change, or if you're ready to delve into planning.

PLANNING AS A PROCESS

Too often planning is thought of as simple problem solving—the client has a problem, and with a good plan, he or she can solve it. From this perspective, planning becomes about lists, tasks, and schedules. The person is lost. Motivation is assumed, and therefore secondary. But this is not how planning should be, for that type of planning is a roll of the dice, with success left to chance. Instead, you want to increase the odds of success. In MI, the goal is to be with the person as he or she develops a plan. It is not to develop the plan for them. The spirit of MI is still present throughout this final stage. You are a partner, a collaborator, and one who understands. Your empathy and acceptance help the client see the road ahead (and its obstacles) more clearly. To do this, you need a map of your own. A good guide knows a bit about what lies ahead, even if the map is incomplete or if the ultimate travel decisions are not yours to make.

Think again of our map, with X marking the spot. Planning is about how one reaches that spot. There are three possible scenarios for you and your offender client as you consider how to best reach your intended end point. In one, the clearest and most direct route is obvious. In another, there are several paths, and together you must choose the best one. And in still another, while the end goal is obvious, you and the client are unsure of how to reach it. Let us consider each in turn.

Scenario 1: The Obvious Path

The offender knows where he or she needs to go. You wholeheartedly agree. What's more, you both clearly see how to get there. What could go wrong? Lest you think you have no role in this scenario, remember that things do not always go as planned, and it also helps to have your directions written out beforehand. After all, sometimes one begins a journey and then loses the map, loses signal on the trusty GPS, encounters detours that necessitate additional help, or becomes tired and simply stops. To help with this, you first summarize the anticipated plan. Summaries remain important, even after the processes of engaging, focusing, and evoking. As you continue your conversation, summarize what the offender has said about specific elements that begin to form the plan: "You see yourself getting there by finding a therapist, keeping a schedule, and figuring out when you're stressed and might want to call your former dealer. And it's important that you talk to people who are supportive of you, like your mother and your girlfriend, in the meantime. They keep you motivated."

Be watchful for opportunities to further elicit mobilizing change talk. The summary above hints at occasions to take steps or evoke activation and commitment language. Imagine adding questions intended to elicit such talk more directly: "How ready are you to find a therapist to help you?"; "What would be a first step in talking to your mother and your girlfriend about what you need right now?"; "How might you go about recognizing those moments when you are likely to contact your former dealer?" Such questions not only invite mobilizing change talk but also strengthen the offender's awareness of components of the emerging plan. This technique may similarly introduce chances for troubleshooting. Perhaps the client realizes during this exchange that while his mother is supportive, she isn't able to help him in the way that he needs. Best for this to surface now, rather than after the offender has built her into his plan in a way that might not be successful. While troubleshooting, focusing on solutions rather than dwelling on problems will help the client avoid lapsing into sustain talk. Further, ensuring that the offender is generating solutions to the problems avoids falling into the expert trap, where the client describes problems and you solve them.

Finally, even though there seems to be a clear path, the offender will need to make things more specific moving forward. This may include identifying intermediary steps or different mechanisms for monitoring progress and making adjustments along the way. For example, the offender who knows he or she must find a therapist will need to identify therapists who are available and who provide the type of treatment needed, as well as decide how they will pay for sessions.

Scenario 2: There Are Several Clear Paths

Oftentimes, there may be multiple ways of reaching the same intended goal. When this occurs, the process of planning involves prioritizing a path and choosing the one that seems to best fit the offender's needs and resources. Using our hypothetical client John, imagine the options available to him to improve his mood. One method might involve finding ways to reduce his overall stress level, presupposing his mood swings and low mood are exacerbated by the stress in his life. Another path would be to seek therapy, or even the help of medications. Still another might be to begin taking better care of himself through diet and exercise to reduce his vulnerability to strong emotion and foster healthy life choices. Alternatively, he could pursue all three, though it might be overwhelming for him to do so while he's facing urges for substance use, seeking a new job, and trying to repair his relationship with his wife and children.

Again, there are several steps to help select the most compelling alternative. First, re-identify the goal. Though the goal was set through the process of focusing, it is possible that the goal has become less clear, or that other, related goals are currently muddying the water, so to speak. A reminder of what the goal is can assist in clarifying the best path. Second, it is helpful to list the potential options. As with agenda mapping, one can map various paths (Miller & Rollnick, 2013). This may include information that the offender has already provided, or with permission, you may suggest potential routes that you know of based on previous experience with other clients, or your professional knowledge and training. Third, not all options may be appealing, available, or realistic, so you can simply ask the client for his or her preferences. Also, the client may inherently know that some paths are more likely to be successful than others. This may be based on prior experience or so-called "gut feeling." Our offender, John, may simply know that physical limitations prohibit exercise routines he would most enjoy. Or that his insurance plan is more likely to cover the cost of medication than additional therapy. The final strategies are to summarize what seems to emerge as the best path, and to troubleshoot potential obstacles that may arise.

Scenario 3: Creating a Path

As you can well imagine, there are times when the client responds to the key question with "I don't know." Hearing "I'm not sure" or "I don't know" is certainly frustrating. You may think, "How could you *not* know? We've been talking about it forever!" We live in a culture that rewards the correct answer—it does not reward saying, "I'm confused and unsure." When faced with this response from your client, instead ask for elaboration: "Tell me more about that."; "We've talked about several issues—what part of this are you unsure about?" For instance, John presents to his case manager or his probation officer with a need to address his substance abuse problem. However, he must also address underlying difficulties with his mood, problems in his relationship, lack of consistent employment, and other life stressors. He is also under supervision from the court, which imposes additional restrictions on his behavior and requirements he must meet. It may therefore be very realistic that he doesn't know how to reach the goals he has set for himself. When a client is unsure or confused, remember to slow down, ask for elaboration, and break things into more manageable chunks.

The danger when an offender client says, "I don't know" is the temptation to simply adopt a directing style and tell the offender what to do. In some cases, the offender even expects you to do this. Again, the spirit of MI can guide your reply: "I've got some ideas, but first let's take a look at your thoughts." Don't give in too easily, but rather allow the plan to continue in a collaborative fashion, with you as a guide to help navigate the way, evoking the offender's own strengths, ideas and experiences. Much like having multiple paths from which to choose, when there is no predetermined path, first confirm the goal. It is then helpful to brainstorm with the client possible options for reaching that goal. What has worked in the past? What else has the person tried before? Even if previous attempts at change were unsuccessful, the strategies the client used then may still be viable for future attempts. Thinking aloud about possibilities can generate a list of potential options, from which you can then continue the steps outlined above in Scenario 2. Let us take a look at a brief example of what this might look like with our hypothetical offender John, in Box 11.1. John and his case manager begin with re-creating solutions that helped him in the past, followed by a summary that culminates with John identifying his preferences for a workable plan. Beyond that, he and his case manager would likely go into greater detail regarding the proposed plan and troubleshoot potential obstacles. With any of the scenarios, the goal is to develop a thorough and targeted plan for a specific outcome that has been agreed upon by you and the client, and that also satisfies important elements of the offender's court or agency requirements.

> *The danger when an offender client says, "I don't know" is the temptation to simply adopt a directing style and tell the offender what to do.*

ROADBLOCKS IN CREATING A PLAN

Using our earlier example of climbing a hill, with preparatory change talk being the trek up the mighty slope and mobilizing change talk being the rapid descent toward the bottom, we may all too often think of planning as the welcoming plain at the bottom—free of rocks or debris and easily traversed. However, sometimes there are obstacles that can interfere with a smooth transition from evoking to developing a plan, many of which are particularly evident with offenders.

One such challenge can be the involvement of others. As is briefly referenced by John in Box 11.1, he may not have full ability to choose his own therapist. Clients who include mental health, offender-specific, or substance-related treatment as part of their plan may be restricted to only certain providers—not all mental health professionals are able to provide offender-specific services (e.g., sex offender treatment, domestic violence family reunification), or are comfortable working within the context of court-ordered treatment. Relatedly, some case managers, community supervisors, or residential (i.e., correctional or inpatient)

BOX 11.1. CREATING A PLAN WITH JOHN

JOHN: I really want to get my mood under control. I know that when I'm down or angry, I'm most likely to turn to drugs. But I don't know what I need to do next.

CASE MANAGER: Well, let's think about it. You want to improve your mood, or your ability to handle your mood?

JOHN: Oh, my ability to handle it, I guess. I don't want to feel sad or angry, but that's probably just part of life. But I would like to cope with it better.

CASE MANAGER: Okay. You said before that you've done therapy in the past. What was that like?

JOHN: It worked for a little while. Parts of it were helpful. But then I got cocky, I think, and I started thinking I could do it on my own, and that I didn't need to tell someone about my problems in order to fix them. It started to feel like a waste of time.

CASE MANAGER: What was helpful about it?

JOHN: I liked the therapist. She was easy for me to talk to. I also liked this workbook she gave me about anger. It made a lot of sense.

CASE MANAGER: You were helped by having a therapist you could talk to, and by having a book that made sense and that you could look at in between sessions. What else has helped you in the past with your mood?

JOHN: Um, this probably sounds silly, but exercise helped. Like if I could just take a walk, or go to the gym on a regular basis, I didn't get so angry all the time. I was probably too tired to! (*Laughs.*)

CASE MANAGER: That makes sense. Exercise helps a lot of people, I think. And you enjoyed it.

JOHN: I did. I don't know why I stopped. Probably because I was more concerned about getting high.

CASE MANAGER: You wish you could get back into it.

JOHN: I do. I haven't thought about that in a long time. And also, I did take some medications for a while. An antidepressant. I stopped because I couldn't afford the co-pays. Put the money toward a different drug, you know.

CASE MANAGER: How do you feel about medications now?

JOHN: I'd like to try it without them. I am working so hard to not do drugs. I know it's not the same thing, but I'm really trying to find ways to fix things without meds or drugs.

CASE MANAGER: Okay. Medications are perhaps not the way you want to go this time. What else has helped with your mood?

JOHN: I like spending time with my kids. They are sometimes pretty stressful, you know, but doing fun things with them helps. Makes me forget about

(continued)

BOX 11.1. (*continued*)

---

my problems for a while. Oh, and when I was in treatment before, my therapist had me keep track of my sleep. I thought about it just now talking about the kids. We were trying to get the youngest on a sleep schedule, and my therapist talked about how even adults need a regular sleep schedule too, and how it helps with your mood.

CASE MANAGER: You put a lot of work into this in the past. You went to therapy, which you found helpful because of the therapist and the workbook. You don't like the idea, though, of taking medications—at least not now. You enjoyed spending time with your kids, and it helped improve your mood. Another thing was your self-care routine. Getting regular sleep and exercise helped you to feel better. Have I left anything out?

JOHN: No, that sounds right.

CASE MANAGER: Good. Now, what's your sense of which of these options might work best in your current situation?

JOHN: Um, I'm not sure. They all sound good. Well, some are better than others. Like right now, I don't have a job yet and I need to be completely flexible so that I don't have anything standing in my way when they call me about a job interview or want to schedule me for work. So that might make an exercise routine tough. I might start it and then have to quit, and that wouldn't help me much.

CASE MANAGER: Okay. Exercise might not be the best bet right now.

JOHN: I have to see a therapist. That's in my court program. But I can talk about my problems with anger and depression with the same therapist they're giving me for substance abuse issues. And really, I want to spend more time with my kids. This last arrest really made me scared I would lose them. So I think those two things are really the way I need to go.

---

supervisors may desire involvement in the development and approval of the plan. This could range from simply having input, to determining steps toward addressing the offender's needs, to involvement as a co-facilitator in therapeutic groups (a highly controversial issue; e.g., McGrath, Cumming, & Holt, 2002). Depending on the circumstances, judges or supervisory bodies may request some degree of oversight and approval of the offender's plan. All such actions limit the autonomy that is so critical to MI.

What to do? MI would not have you blindly fight the system, nor would it recommend ignoring the centrality of client autonomy. One important strategy is to simply acknowledge the client's bind. Using reflections and accurate empathy may help problem-solve potential disagreements or resolve negative feelings that result from the involvement of these additional parties without becoming mired in the sense of unfairness or defiance that may lead offenders to circumvent effective planning.

Another challenge is lack of resources that offenders may face as they attempt to develop and implement a plan. For some, employment options may be limited due to the nature of their convictions. For others, restrictions in transportation (e.g., suspended driver's license) or residence (e.g., restrictions for sex offenders in the United States) may impact their intended plans for change. Similarly, restitution or fines may take priority over providing additional monies for their family or the cost of educational programs to better themselves and their vocational options. For those in residential, inpatient, or correctional settings, the staff or particular treatment options they identify as important to part of their rehabilitation may be less available or contingent on other factors beyond their control, such as time to release or policy-driven qualifications for such programming. Finally, for offenders involved in court-ordered intensive programming, there may not be enough hours in the day to incorporate other elements of the plan. For example, those in intensive outpatient or day treatment programs may already face 3 to 4 hours a day of structured programming, in addition to work and reporting requirements. Finding time to incorporate other, more individualized elements of the plan may not be possible.

Again, understanding and transparent responses go a long way with such clients. Limitations and restrictions are a reality for many offenders, and they can interfere with motivation as well as the implementation of a desired plan. A first step is to simply acknowledge the struggle and empathize with the offender—it seems like an insurmountable hurdle in the face of so many needed changes that must occur, despite the fact that such obstacles (such as intensive programming) are actually intended to help rather than hinder behavior change. Another strategy is to encourage clients to incorporate such limitations or resource deficiencies into their planning. Preplanning around such obstacles may increase a sense of self-efficacy and circumvent the potential derailment of an otherwise workable plan. It will also increase the likelihood that clients will actively problem-solve with you or involved others as additional problems arise. They will already have experience talking through such challenges.

A final issue to consider with offenders is that they may falter in their confidence and commitment as they become overwhelmed with the enormity of all that lies before them. Even when there's a map, it can seem like a distant destination or a daunting road ahead. Affirmations and continued efforts to strengthen commitment and confidence can help.

MAINTAINING COMMITMENT AND REINFORCING CHANGE

What happens when the offender leaves your office, plan in hand? The work of MI would appear to be over. However, this is not so. Many who work with offenders are familiar with the experience of helping them develop a plan—a plan that they fully intend to implement and feel is best for them—but still feeling apprehensive. The plan may not work. The offender may falter in his or her commitment. Unexpected setbacks will inevitably occur, regardless of how much you and the client may have anticipated them. And of greatest concern, changes that the offender has successfully made might not receive the positive feedback and support needed to maintain long-term efforts at behavior change. Such occurrences are disappointing, certainly. They do not suggest, however, that the work of MI was in vain. Instead, they perhaps suggest that the work of MI should continue so as to maintain commitment and further reinforce initial signs of change. In other words, planning is not a singular, one-time event that ends your relationship with the offender, or the work of change.

Strengthening Commitment

In Chapters 9 and 10 we described recognizing commitment language and responding to it in a way that moves the client closer to change. Now, we consider other aspects of commitment that go beyond the process of evoking. At that point, it was largely you and the client exploring the client's reasons for change and steps to initiate the change process. But it is not always just about the client's commitment alone. With offenders, as with other clients, it is important to consider the role of others in furthering the client's motivation and commitment to change.

See, for example, a follow-up appointment with John in Box 11.2. Notice how the conversation progresses. John has initiated change. He has a therapist, and he is working on his depression. He has a job. But he recognizes that his wife might be doubtful of his ability to change, even despite his recent efforts to make a difference. The case manager uses a combination of skillful, complex reflections to help John consider how

BOX 11.2. JOHN DESCRIBES HIS WIFE'S INVOLVEMENT IN HIS CHANGE PLAN

CASE MANAGER: I haven't seen you in a few months. How is it going?

JOHN: Okay, I guess. I was able to get in to see a therapist who is helping me with my depression. I really feel like I can talk with her. It's helped.

CASE MANAGER: Good, good. Your depression feels more under control.

JOHN: Yeah, I guess. I hope I can keep it up.

CASE MANAGER: You're worried.

JOHN: Well, there's just a lot going on. I'm glad I have a therapist. I have a job, though it's not really the best. But it is a job, for the time being. I can live with that. My wife still gets on my case a lot. It's like I'm not making progress fast enough for her.

CASE MANAGER: She doesn't see yet how the plan works.

JOHN: Yeah, I guess that's it. She doesn't really know much about the plan. She knows there is one. I mean, I did tell her I was going to therapy, and she was good with that.

CASE MANAGER: How does she feel about you being in therapy?

JOHN: I guess she is skeptical. I've been in therapy before. I could see then how it helped, but because I kept getting into trouble, maybe she didn't see it in the same way I did. And all she knows right now is that I'm trying to do the right thing, and that I meet with a therapist.

CASE MANAGER: What would happen if you talked to her about it in more detail?

JOHN: I don't know. I guess I figured she wouldn't want to know that much about it. But maybe she does. She always asks when I get back how I'm doing, and if all of this is helping. It is, and like I said, I can see it, but I don't really give her much to go on. And if I did tell her about it, it might make her feel better. And it might hold me more accountable to really staying the course.

CASE MANAGER: I think you're right.

---

talking about his change plan with his wife might solidify his commitment and also engender her support.

Making a commitment known to others has several effects. First, it may communicate to persons who are less invested in the offender's change (e.g., friends who continue to use drugs or engage in other illegal behaviors) that the offender intends to behave in a different way. Their reaction to such information will alert the offender to potential roadblocks. We can well imagine that friends and family who are dismissive of the offender's commitment would thus communicate that they may stand in the way of change. Another effect of verbalizing commitment to others is that it strengthens resolve to be successful. Making others aware of a planned change increases accountability. If you don't follow through, then you have to explain yourself later. And at times, the avoidance of such an explanation can be a powerful motivator. Most people would rather talk about their successes than their failures.

Letting others know about a planned change directly is one strategy. Another is to self-monitor, which is a common technique in many therapies and other strategies for change. Keeping track of important elements of the plan—number of job applications submitted, times when urges to use substances are the strongest, or rating anger during different times of the day—can not only bolster commitment in small ways but can also alert the client to times when his or her behavior may deviate from the planned course. Relatedly, the client may enlist others in monitoring practices. John, for example, could ask his wife to rate how she perceives his level of depression during the week, which will keep him talking about important elements of his mood improvement plan, give him valuable feedback, and reinforce important changes that he does make. All of these can be useful in strengthening John's commitment to continue working on the problem.

Supporting Change

As we have noted throughout this text, offenders often face very complex changes. Seldom is there only *one* thing that needs to be addressed. Such complexity can lead them to feel discouraged as they implement the plan. Perhaps the road is long, and they become tired. Or the road simply leads to other roads, and they become impatient with being so far from the end goal. By supporting change, you reinforce their persistence as they stay the course.

The same elements of MI that helped you reach this point with your client can help support the offender's efforts to maintain early change. A collaborative partnership with compassion and accurate empathy helps maintain a strong relationship. This relationship is reinforcing in itself. Humans are social animals. We want to know what others think of us. In particular, we want to know what others think when they matter in some way. Having a strong continued relationship offers support and facilitates further change. Similarly, the skills you used to engage the offender (i.e., OARS) are also useful in supporting change. Asking open questions shows interest in how the client is implementing the change plan. Affirmations, by their very nature, are supportive. Reflect and summarize important steps toward change. Having clients' efforts noticed and reflected helps them recognize their progress. This is important, as sometimes people lose sight of all they have done when they are in the midst of doing it.

Other components of MI can also help. As important milestones in the plan are met, goals and priorities evolve. It may be useful to refocus and shift the planned destination. Once people have begun to make a change, they may recognize other needed changes, or rediscover others that are now more important. This is natural and should not be viewed as reluctance to address the "real" problem, failure to prioritize the plan, or lack of commitment. Instead, it may reflect insight into the nature of the offender's problems, as well as an important step in the person's growth. After all, the ultimate goal is to help the offender client make changes but to also make them sustainable. Sustainability comes from the individual's own ability to assess the situation, recognize the problem, and initiate adjustments accordingly. Once again, using open questions, reflections, and strategies like agenda mapping and the importance ruler can facilitate this process.

Finally, as a form of support, you may be called upon to remind the client of the goal. This is particularly needed when the client seems discouraged or doubtful of his or her chances of success. This involves re-evoking change talk, eliciting commitment language, and addressing sustain talk in a way that acknowledges realistic barriers to success in the offender's environment. The need for change talk is continuous, and it doesn't simply end once early signs of change have occurred. Our offender John has identified seeing a therapist as part of his plan to work on his depression and anger, which will in turn influence his need to use substances to control and mask his moods. He has found a therapist, yet he still has work to do in treatment. Thus, while it was first necessary to elicit change talk and strengthen commitment to attending therapy, evoking change talk to see him through the difficult work of therapy remains necessary even beyond early treatment sessions.

Planning can feel quite rewarding after the difficult work of engaging the client, focusing on a relevant goal, and evoking talk that motivates change. In working with offenders, the plan involves many different people, agencies, and efforts. It can be a challenge to coordinate these disparate elements into a workable plan. Even more so, it may be difficult to build in a sense of sustainability and self-sufficiency so that the offender can implement the plan with support and guidance (and without needing directiveness). It is our goal for you to reach this milestone with each of your clients and contribute to lasting behavior change.

CHAPTER 12

RESISTANCE REEXAMINED

There is little evidence for the belief that if you can make them
feel bad enough, they will change.
　　　　　　　　　　—VIETS, WALKER, AND MILLER (2002)

Offender work largely defines "resistance" as any apparent client movement away from change. Resistant clients—whether resisting treatment,
resisting change, or just expressing normal doubt—are quickly labeled
as difficult and intractable. An offender wanting to avoid such a label
must quickly yield to agents of the system. How much and how quickly
the offender must surrender is often subjective. Some require the offender
to capitulate by both agreeing with the other person's view (i.e., "You're
right. I need to . . . ") and demonstrating behavioral compliance. Others
are willing to forgo a conforming attitude in favor of the desired behavior (i.e., "Well, I don't want to, but I'll do it"). In more extreme cases,
offender agency staff expect the offender to "knuckle under"* or offer
a complete submission of will, demonstrated by subservient compliance.
There exists a smaller minority of persons working with offenders who,
even in the face of compliance and a good attitude, will still withhold civil
conversation—refusing to even shake hands with the offender—until the
person has earned dismissal from court jurisdiction (Clark, 2005).

　　This one-sided view of resistance places the locus of responsibility solely on the offender. The person is "difficult" as part of his or

---

* In Dyche and Pardon's 1740 *A Dictionary of All the Words Commonly Us'd in the Eng-
lish Tongue,* this term was defined as "Knuckle or knuckle down: to stoop, bend, yield,
comply with, or submit to." It communicated the act of stooping with one's knuckles low
down or on the ground.

her character. Even when such resistance is viewed as arising from a lifetime of miserable experiences, the concept of resistance nevertheless focuses on the offender's individual character. The interpersonal aspects of interactions with an offender are vastly underemphasized. In their early work with MI (see Miller & Rollnick, 1991), resistance was viewed as the product of, or at least highly responsive to, *the style of interaction*. In other words, what we traditionally have called the offender's "resistance" actually exists only in the context of a given interaction or relationship.

Persons who work with offenders are relentlessly plagued by this "resistance." Yet much of what we have already presented describes resistance as an interaction. The righting reflex (Chapter 4), the many interviewing traps that inhibit engagement (Chapter 4), overuse of a directive style (Chapter 4), and not listening or distracted half listening (Chapter 3) only make matters worse. MI finds no merit in assigning blame—whether it be directed toward the offender or toward those who work with them. In this chapter we reexamine this resistance within the context of sustain talk and discord, additionally considering the role of sanctions and violations in the spirit of MI.

REEXAMINING RESISTANCE

The idea of resistance is that a person is actively working against something, or providing pushback that is intended to derail or stop forward movement. In her work examining the back-and-forth of snippets of MI, Moyers (from her work on Moyers & Martin, 2006; T. B. Miller, personal communication, September 16–17, 2013) noted that in many cases what was being called "resistance" was simply sustain talk. There is nothing inherently pathological or oppositional about sustain talk; it's simply one side of a person's ambivalence.

However, while both change and sustain talk are naturally intermingled during the exploration of ambivalence, when pressed by others to change, people naturally voice their sustain talk. With offenders, you may find yourself reacting strongly to sustain talk and making more of it than it is: "He said he doesn't see anything wrong with continuing to inject heroin!"; "She's completely resistant to treatment—she says she could never go to group!"; "This guy says what he does in his home is none of the court's business!" Perhaps due to the extremity and illegality of the behaviors in question, sustain talk from offenders provokes a strong reaction, and is thus more readily labeled as resistance and made part of the offender's problem. Unfortunately, such a reaction will likely strengthen sustain talk and create more pushback from the client.

So if we subtract sustain talk from the larger body of resistance, what is left? Disagreement, not being "on the same wavelength," talking at cross-purposes, or problems in the relationship may be evident. These characterize *discord*. You experience discord, for example, when a client argues with, interrupts, ignores, discounts, or dismisses you. How can you tell the difference between sustain talk and discord? Discord reflects tension, hostility, or dissonance in the alliance. Discord is more about you and the relationship, whereas sustain talk is about the target behavior or change (e.g., "I want to keep using heroin"). Discord is like a fire—or at least, smoke—in the helping relationship. What's more, it's a sign that the conversation has become more about you, and the relationship, than the offender's process of change. Let us examine each of these, and what to do with them, more closely.

SUSTAIN TALK

Sustain talk reflects only one side of the offender's ambivalence. As with change talk, it cannot occur unless the offender first knows what the change goal is. By nature then, it identifies a focus. Sustain talk supports:

- *Keeping the status quo*: "I want to keep dealing drugs" or "I really don't see anything wrong with keeping things the way they are now."
- *Assessing the status quo as acceptable or good*: "I like the easy money from dealing drugs" or "Sometimes when I show a little muscle, even if it hurts someone, they give me more respect."
- *Considering change as bad or something to avoid*: "Work a 40-hour-a-week job? That's not for me" or "People won't respect me if I walk away from a fight."

Don't assume that the presence of sustain talk means that there is no recognition of a need for change. Such an assumption may drive your response to be the righting reflex (Chapter 3) or a directive style, neither of which will be particularly beneficial to the conversation. These techniques can quickly turn sustain talk into discord. Nevertheless, sustain talk matters. The more people verbalize and explore sustain talk, the more they talk themselves out of change. Thus, while it reflects a normal part of ambivalence, gradually increasing the ratio of change talk to sustain talk will further the conversation.

How does this look in practice? *Change talk* reflects the pros of change, and the cons of the status quo. *Sustain talk* reflects the opposite: the pros of the status quo and the cons of change. Early on, the two may be evenly balanced in a 1:1 ratio, which is one working definition of ambivalence. The cons of change may even outweigh the pros, particularly in the beginning of the conversation. As you proceed with MI, change talk typically increases, whereas sustain talk diminishes, so that later change talk statements may counterbalance sustain talk by 2:1 or more. That is the trajectory of a conversation associated with subsequent behavior change. The shifting balance of sustain talk to change talk predicts the likelihood of change, and you can influence that balance. If you elicit a lot of "resistance"—sustain talk and discord—change is unlikely to happen. The goal is to help offenders talk *themselves* into changing.

So pay attention to sustain talk, recognizing it for what it is—just one side of ambivalence. And also notice what may be more accurately described as discord as a signal of dissonance in your collaborative relationship. These are not character defects of the client; they are normal dynamics in any conversation about change. The next step is then to use the strategies for responding to sustain talk and eliciting further change talk that were described more fully in Chapter 10.

> *The shifting balance of sustain talk to change talk predicts the likelihood of change, and you can influence that balance.*

DISCORD

Now we turn to discord, or a signal of disharmony in your collaborative relationship. Once again, discord is a sign that there is a problem brewing between you and the offender, rather than a defect in the offender or in his or her motivation for change. What are the signs of something smoldering in your working alliance? Think of these as *smoke alarms,* or a call that alerts you to nearby danger and prompts you to recognize signs of conflict in the relationship.

Smoke Alarm 1: Defending

You know something is amiss when the client feels a need to defend him- or herself. This can take many forms:

- Dishonesty—"I didn't do it."
- Blaming—"It's not my fault."
- Consensus—"Everyone does it."
- Intention—"I didn't mean to do it."
- Minimizing—"It's not that bad."
- Justification—"I needed the money."

While on the surface these are about "it"—the change target—and thus overlap with sustain talk, these statements also have a definite overlay of defending one's integrity, autonomy, normality, or self-esteem. People defend, of course, in response to perceived attack or threat. Signs like these communicate that the offender is feeling personally threatened.

Given that many offenders do feel as if they are trapped by a system that expects them to fail, it is not surprising that a certain percentage may be deceptive or defensive in order to win over the system or increase their chances of benefit. At the same time, most offenders bend the truth or justify their behaviors for pretty ordinary reasons. It is not so much the presence or absence of these defending behaviors but their degree of seriousness and pervasiveness that becomes a problem.

Defending involves two types of dishonesty. One is intentional and largely self-aware, though it may also involve some degree of self-deception. People tend to assume two things about themselves (Sigmon & Snyder 1993): "I'm a good person" and "I am in control most of the time." These assumptions are self-protective and drive us to defend ourselves in certain ways. For instance, a person will be deliberately dishonest to save face. This maintains a positive self-image. Similarly, a person will defend to save face for someone he or she cares about. Relationships are powerful motivators. Abused children may lie to protect their parent(s), or family members may willingly lie about behaviors they still do not condone. And also, a person will be dishonest to prevent a perceived loss of freedom or resources. This one is particularly relevant for offenders. There are penalties for admitting law-breaking behavior, and an offender must weigh the immediate penalties resulting from telling the truth against the possibly worse, but less certain, penalties that might occur if he or she told a lie. In fact, defending can be a good gamble if the immediate penalties are more certain and possibly just as bad.

There are also deceptive tendencies that are more implicit and may operate somewhat beyond the offender's conscious awareness. People distort information to make it more consistent with their feelings and beliefs (Saarni & Lewis, 1993). People often reinterpret information to make it fit with their basic assumptions about their goodness or competency. Nowhere is this more evident than in making excuses. For example, an offender who believes herself to be generally competent but who has been unsuccessful in sustaining employment may blame the circumstances or her supervisor. A person may also distort information based on who is asking the question, or how it is phrased. Asking, for example, "Why didn't you . . . ?" prompts a list of excuses—often excuses that maintain self-image or autonomy.

Smoke Alarm 2: Squaring Off

A sure sign of fire in the working alliance is an oppositional stance, which signals that you are perceived as an adversary rather than an advocate. These have more of a "you" quality to them:

> "*You* don't care about me."
> "Who are *you* to tell me what to do?"
> "*You* don't know what you're talking about."
> "*You* have no idea what it's like for me."
> "*You're* wrong about that."
> "*You* don't know that."

Here is an invitation to a power struggle, inviting an argument or efforts to persuade the offender to see your point of view. Because the topic of conversation is personal change, however, the client holds most of the power.

Smoke Alarm 3: Interrupting

Another sign of discord is when a client talks over you, interrupting while you are speaking. The occurrence of interrupting, rather than the content that has been interrupted, is the signal. What might this communicate? "You don't understand"; "You're not hearing me"; "You're talking too much"; "Listen to me"; "I don't agree with you."

For some, this emerges as a characteristic style of their speech—if they do listen at all, it is just long enough to decide what to say next, and then they begin talking. But also consider that it may be a sign of discord, particularly if the prior rhythm of the conversation has suddenly changed.

Smoke Alarm 4: Disengagement

A fourth smoke alarm is when the client disengages from the conversation. The person seems inattentive and distracted, or simply ignores you. Perhaps the client changes the subject and goes off on a tangent. Her eyes glaze over, or you find her glancing at the clock. This may mean any number of things, ranging from unwillingness to continue the conversation to merely becoming inpatient or bored with a topic they would rather be done exploring.

Why is discord a concern? Some might regard signals like this to be a good sign that you are "getting to them." Discord is a concern, however, because it signals a breakdown in the working alliance and is inversely related to subsequent change (Miller et al., 1993; Patterson & Chamberlain, 1994; Safran, Crocker, McMain, & Murray, 1990). It's not just that "difficult people don't change." The amount of discord is a product of interaction; you can influence both discord and change.

We also hasten to add that signs of discord are culturally relative. What signals a breakdown of collaboration in one culture or subculture (e.g., lack of eye contact) may not be important in another. This can be a problem when counseling across cultural differences, where reflection is a particularly good tool to check on meaning.

YOUR OWN CONTRIBUTION TO DISCORD

Until now, we have largely explored discord from the perspective or behavior exhibited by the offender. But it is important to remember that discord can also arise as the result of your mood or approach. It is more likely to occur when you are feeling tired, under stress or distracted, or even just very motivated to help someone solve an urgent problem. Perhaps you stop listening, or your righting reflex twitches. You begin arguing for change and providing solutions, elicit natural pushback from the offender, and the rapport between you is in jeopardy. See a brief example below.

> CORRECTIONAL OFFICER: I think it's time for you to take this seriously and do something about it.
>
> OFFENDER: It's just not a priority for me right now. I think I'll be all right.
>
> CORRECTIONAL OFFICER: I have a hard time seeing how you're going to be all right if you don't change anything. You keep on doing the same thing and expect a different result!

OFFENDER: Look, I'm fine. I can take care of myself, okay? I don't need to talk about this with you.

Notice how the discord in this instance also takes the form of sustain talk, and it's clearly not the result of the refined listening that lies at the heart of MI. The correctional officer has become restless to push on and has left the offender behind.

You may notice signals of discord within yourself. Perhaps it's physical—a tight feeling in the stomach, or a flushing in the face. Perhaps it's silent self-talk: "I can't believe she is sitting here and telling me this isn't a problem"; "What's the matter with her?"; "How many times have we talked about this?" You may also feel anxious, wondering what will happen to your client, or if negative outcomes will be seen as your fault. Of course, attending to this internal monologue prevents you from listening to the client.

DISCORD WITHIN THE PROCESSES OF MI

Discord can occur for different reasons across the four processes of MI. Here we present a brief discussion of different contexts in which it may emerge.

Discord in Engaging

Some people are angry and defensive before the conversation even begins. Discord can thus emerge quite early as an obstacle to engagement. This may be the product of prior experiences with coercion, unfair expectations, or poor conduct from others. MI is a particularly effective approach for working with people who are angry and defensive at the outset (Karno & Longabaugh, 2004; Waldron, Miller, & Tonigan, 2001). The good news is that change is predicted not by the offender's initial level of commitment but rather by the pattern of change in motivation over the course of the MI session (Amrhein, et al., 2003). You may not responsible for the client's starting point, but you do have considerable influence over what happens next.

There are many factors that can promote client disengagement. It's not unheard of for an initial interview to fall right into an assessment trap: "Thanks for coming in. Let's get started. I need to ask you some questions, and you just tell me 'yes' or 'no.'" With this approach, disengagement, passivity, and discord seem assured.

One can unwittingly contribute to discord in more subtle ways as well. Labeling and blaming (see Chapter 4) promote distancing. For example, when interviewing someone who drinks too much, use of the term "alcoholic" may generate discord almost immediately, and it can be a challenge to reengage. Even the language of having "a problem" can quickly evoke defensiveness.

Discord in Focusing

Discord can also arise during focusing as disagreements about what to discuss and targets for change emerge. At the outset, a person may have multiple concerns, and as we've noted, what is on your mind as a critical area of concern might not be his or her highest priority. The premature focus trap, or pushing too soon for a change target that the offender does not yet share, can create discord at this stage. In an offender treatment program for women, for example, the staff may find that clients have some concerns about their drug use or other illegal behaviors, but these may feel less pressing (to the offender) than problems like finding a job, housing, child care, and personal safety. A single-minded focus on one problem is likely to undermine a good working alliance and foster discord.

Discord in Evoking

There's no single dividing line between sustain talk and discord. If you have successfully engaged well with an offender and have an agreed focus, sustain talk still emerges quite naturally. This need not be viewed as a problem or signal of discord, as sustain talk is a normal part of ambivalence. However, if you push the conversation in a hasty direction, or at too quick a pace, discord may result.

Discord is a common consequence of the righting reflex. Pushing for change elicits a "pushback" from the offender, and this pattern can escalate into a discordant back-and-forth that damages rapport. During the evoking process, discord can also arise from trying to move prematurely into planning. Pushing for a change plan before the client is ready can reverse whatever progress has been made thus far. See below for a brief example.

PROBATION OFFICER: You've told me some reasons why making this change would be a good idea. So what are you actually going to do about it?

OFFENDER: I don't know. I wish I could do something, but it's not so easy.

PROBATION OFFICER: Well, let's just talk about how you could do it. What ideas do you have?

OFFENDER: That's just it. I'm not sure I'm ready for this.

PROBATION OFFICER: How can I help you be more ready? Don't you see the benefits it will bring?

OFFENDER: That's not the point, really. I can see that there could be some benefits, but to be honest, I feel like the court is pushing me into this.

This person is indeed feeling pushed. There is still more work to do with evoking, and the signals are clear. It's just too early to push ahead toward committing to a plan. If the probation officer continues in this manner, there may be some reengaging work to do as well.

Discord in Planning

Finally, discord can arise during the planning process. After successful navigation through engaging, focusing and evoking, it is tempting to think, "Okay, I can take it from here," and then begin telling the client what to do in a directive style. Why not? He or she is ready to plan and problem solve, right? Maybe not. Planning is a collaborative process, and directing instead of guiding can create discord and break down your careful work. In other instances, though you and the offender may agree on the change goal and its importance, discord can arise over the best way to proceed.

RESPONDING TO DISCORD

What all of these potential sources of discord have in common is a breakdown in the dance. Instead of moving and working together, it begins to feel like a struggle, and toes are invariably stepped on. It usually results from a clash between the staff person's righting reflex and the offender's ambivalence. Signs of discord are like a smoke alarm. They are your client telling you not to do more of the same, but to try a different approach.

We now look at how to respond to experiences of discord. While sustain talk is about the problem, discord is about you! Or more accurately, discord is about the current state of your relationship with the offender. In many ways, MI responses to discord resemble how one responds to sustain talk. (We again refer readers to Chapter 10 for a review of those methods.) Reflection remains a key tool for understanding one another and restoring a working alliance.

> OFFENDER: How old are you? How can you possibly understand me?
>
> REFLECTION: You're wondering if I'll really be able to help you.
>
> Or:
>
> AMPLIFIED REFLECTION: It seems like there's no chance at all that I could help you at all.
>
> Or:
>
> DOUBLE-SIDED REFLECTION: You're looking for some help, and you're not really sure if I'm the right person to provide it.
>
> OFFENDER: I'm not going to quit, [sustain talk] and you can't make me. [discord]
>
> REFLECTION: That's right. I know I can't make that decision for you even if I wanted to. [emphasizing autonomy]

In addition to these, there are other ways of responding to discord that can be helpful. One is *apologizing.* When you've stepped on someone's toes, it is polite to say that you're sorry. This costs you nothing and immediately acknowledges the collaborative nature of the relationship: "I'm sorry"; "I must have misunderstood you"; "It sounds like I must have insulted you there"; "I didn't mean to lecture you."

Another is *affirming.* An affirmation can help to heal tension in your working alliance. Sincere affirming aims to diminish defensiveness and reflects a respectful relationship.

> OFFENDER: I can do this on my own without your help!
>
> AFFIRMATION: Once you make your mind up about something, you can get it done.
>
> OFFENDER: You don't know what you're talking about. You don't know me like I know myself.
>
> AFFIRMATION: You've really thought this through.

Another possible response to discord is *shifting focus* away from the hot topic or sore spot, rather than continuing to exacerbate it.

OFFENDER: Are you saying that this is my fault? That I'm not a good husband?

SHIFTING FOCUS: I'm not interested in blaming or name-calling. What matters to me is how you would like your relationship to be better, and how you might get there.

OFFENDER: Do you think I have a drinking problem?

SHIFTING FOCUS: I leave labels to others. What I care about is you and what you think.

There is no single formula for responding to sustain talk and discord. The key is to respond in a collaborative, accepting way that honors autonomy and does not invite defense of the status quo. There are many ways to do this well.

ADDRESSING VIOLATIONS AND SANCTIONS

We noted in Chapter 4 that MI is not a cure-all, quick fix, or magic wand. Even in the best of situations—after deep listening and thoughtful work to start engagement—offenders can make choices and engage in behaviors you wish they wouldn't. Such times do call for a response. Some personnel in offender service agencies may chide, mock, or tease their colleagues who use MI. Such derision may be particularly apparent when violations or sanctions are needed, as they assume practitioners of MI are "against" sanctioning problematic behavior. First, they may mock what they consider to be the "softness" of MI. A gentle rejoinder to this is that MI is neither hard nor soft—it's smart. Better to have a style that functions flexibly in a variety of situations, and that also continues your ability to work effectively with an offender despite setbacks. Second, they may tease you by saying that MI is all-helpful, and that the practitioner of MI will never have to deal with violations or sanctions. Not true. We have never suggested MI is perfect. It is just an advantage. Even with the best application, you may need to address violations and sanctions.

Defending and Dishonesty: What Can Be Done about It?

First, don't take it personally. As we noted earlier, taking full responsibility for negative outcomes can conflict with a person's perceptions of himself or herself as good and in control. With offenders, lying and deception occur not so much to "con" the staff person as to defend these assumptions about themselves—their behavior may be a product of self-deception.

Fortunately, a positive relationship between you and the offender makes lying less probable. Some believe that a confrontational style sends a message that you cannot be fooled or taken in, but the opposite is true—a harsh, coercive style can prompt an offender to lie to save face, and allows the offender to justify his or her dishonesty. Those who have positive, collaborative relationships with offenders are less likely to be lied to. A collaborative working style makes honesty more possible. Rather than ignoring or becoming agitated by deception, an MI approach handles it by taking a step back from the debate.

> *Those who have positive, collaborative relationships with offenders are less likely to be lied to.*

Difficult Situations

When faced with difficult situations, you may be tempted to move to one side or the other—to become too harsh or too friendly—when a more middle-of-the-road approach is appropriate. Correctional staff are like facilitators or consultants in that they manage the relationship between the offender and the court or agency. You do not make decisions for the offender or for the court/agency. You instead view your place as that of a facilitator, allowing you to avoid some of the pitfalls inherent in this dual role. Adopting a middle-of-the-road stance provides the best balance between being an effective advocate for the court/agency and encouraging the offender to make positive changes.

Explaining the Dual Role

You need be up front with offenders about conditions, incentives, and sanctions. You must also be honest with the offender about your dual role as representative and advocate for both the offender and the supervising court or agency. For instance:

> "I want to make you aware that I have a couple of roles here. One of them is to be the court's [facility's] representative and to report your progress on the conditions that they set for you. At the same time, I act on your behalf, to help keep the system off your back and to manage your conditions, while possibly taking some other positive

steps along the way. I'll act as a 'go-between'—that is, between you and the system—but ultimately, you're the one who makes the choices. Tell me how that sounds to you right now. Is there anything you think I need to know before proceeding?"

Being Clear about the Sanctions

You must also ensure that the offender is aware of what sanctions may occur following a violation. This is perhaps most necessary when the offender is close to receiving a sanction. In this example, the offender has shown a significant lack of progress.

> "We've been talking about getting you up to speed on employment. We've been working together for 6 months on this, but it looks like things have been diffcult for you. What happens at this point is that if you can't produce verification of employment by our next meeting, we will move to weekly reporting. That means that instead of meeting once a month, we would meet every week. I know that would make things more diffcult for you, so I guess the ball's in your court. You'll have to decide whether it's easier to make time to do this or whether it's easier to take the sanction. What do you want to do?"

Informing offenders of the sanctions can make compliance more likely, but it is by no means assured. When delivered and described, sanctions should be clear, immediate, and in proportion with the violation. When systems adopt a progressive sanctions model, the incentives and penalties become predictable and apparent to both you and the offender. An offender should never be surprised by a sanction.

Addressing Behavior with a Balanced Attitude

Threatening or criticizing, especially when addressing violations, tends to make diffcult situations worse. An offender may already be defensive about his or her lack of progress, and your agitation or palpable disappointment can make the offender's attitude worse. It's understandable to have emotional investment in how your clients are doing, even if you've only worked with them a short time. If you fall prey to emotional reactivity, it sets the stage for an escalating series of attacks and counterattacks that lead further from change. For this reason, approach violations with a balanced attitude—addressing the behavior and dispensing the appropriate sanction, but not getting agitated or taking the violation personally.

The following dialogue presents a situation in which an offender is getting close to a violation of supervision orders. The case officer describes the consequences but does not get upset by the offender's attitude.

> CASE OFFICER: We've talked about this before. In another 2 weeks, if things are the same as they are now, you will be in violation of this order. We have also talked about how it is up to you. You can certainly ignore the order, but sanctions will be assessed.
>
> OFFENDER: Darn right I can ignore it! This is so stupid!
>
> CASE OFFICER: It seems unfair that you're required to complete this condition. It feels like it might be a waste of your time.
>
> OFFENDER: Yeah, I can't believe I have to do this!
>
> CASE OFFICER: Even though it's hard to swallow, I want to make you aware of what will happen if you don't complete this. If it's not done in the next 2 weeks, you will have to start reporting to me weekly instead of monthly. I guess you have to decide whether it's easier to do it, even though it seems like it might be a waste of your time, or whether it's just easier report to me more often.
>
> OFFENDER: You don't have to report this.
>
> CASE OFFICER: Unfortunately, I do. That's part of my job.
>
> OFFENDER: You mean you can't just let it go?
>
> CASE OFFICER: No, I don't have a choice. But you have a choice, even if I don't. I'm wondering what we can do to help you succeed here?
>
> OFFENDER: I'll think about it. It just seems unfair.

In this example, the case officer refuses to leave the middle, neither defending the order nor siding with the offender to stop the sanction. Some may believe in using a confrontational approach, but at this point, it is probably more appropriate simply to recognize the offender's reluctance and describe what is likely to happen. Regarding the specific sanction, the case officer defers to the system and emphasizes the collaborative relationship between officer and offender. This neutral stance improves the likelihood that a positive decision will eventually overtake the emotions of the moment. Finally, the staff person emphasizes the offender's autonomy and personal responsibility. A probationer on supervision does not have to complete the supervision conditions; taking the sanction always remains an option.

The following dialogue illustrates another diffcult situation—when a violation has seemingly occurred but is denied by the offender. In this example, the case manager presents the results, refuses to defend the lab results, and immediately emphasizes the probationer's autonomy and personal responsibility.

> CASE MANAGER: We got the results of your last drug screen, and it came up positive for methamphetamine. Tell me what happened.
>
> OFFENDER: Positive? Are you sure? It must have been from that last time . . . what was it . . . 3 months ago?
>
> CASE MANAGER: Sort of a mystery as to how it came up positive.
>
> OFFENDER: Yeah, I haven't used, so your lab must have made a mistake.
>
> CASE MANAGER: Unfortunately, the system goes strictly off the results of the screen, so there's nothing we can do about that. But you do have a couple of options at this point. It looks like there will be some jail time, but you also have the option of signing a voluntary admittance. It's a good-faith gesture, and sometimes the judge will be a little more lenient if he or she feels that the person is taking this seriously. It might mean that you could do some sort of drug treatment in lieu of jail time. On the other hand, if you decide that's not something you want, the decision will be based on the results of the drug test, which will probably mean serving time in jail. But again, it's up to you.

The case manager bases his or her decision on the physical evidence rather than on the offender's admission or refusal of drug use. This is also the approach to take when offenders exhibit "pseudocompliance," or talking about change but showing a significant lack of progress. You can provide opportunities for offenders to talk and think about change but still assess the offender's progress in meeting the conditions of supervision or other systemic goals.

Adopting a new approach like MI is a process. Even after initial training, some clients fall back on old habits when violations occur. If the offender shows lack of progress, a common temptation is to switch to more demanding strategies to relieve frustration. However, enforcing sanctions does not require switching to a more heavy-handed style. You can enforce orders and assess sanctions without leaving motivational strategies behind.

The goal is to avoid both the hard and soft approaches. The hard approach is overly directive, defending the court's or agency's authority: "Don't blame the court. You're the one who broke the law." Less examined, but also concerning, is the soft approach, or when you refuse to address violations in order to preserve the relationship: "I won't tell this time, but don't do it again." A positive working alliance with the offender is not the same as ignoring violations. The optimal approach is not the same as the easier approach. We can collaborate with an offender and respect personal choice while still being true to our agency roles.

When the Offender Denies the Initial Offense

Another diffcult situation occurs when the offender denies committing the initial offense. This differs from our scenario above in which an offender has denied a more recent infraction or violation. Rather, the offender may deny the initial charges or conviction and hence feel no need to change. In this situation, some assume that no progress can be made unless the offender first admits the offense.

The first strategy is to avoid defending the court, your agency, the police report, test results, or other decisions or evidentiary proof. If you are willing to view your role as a facilitator rather than an interrogator, a middle way appears. Regardless of the type of agency in which you work, your role is to assist the offender in successfully navigating the system. After you have fulfilled your responsibilities, the choices are still the offender's. This may operate independently of what the offender verbalizes about his or her acceptance of behavior, rules, conditions, judgments, and the like. Although it is best that the offender take responsibility for his or her past actions, admission of guilt need not always be a prerequisite of a change-focused conversation.

> PROBATION OFFICER: So, because your girlfriend said it happened, things looked pretty stacked against you, and you didn't want to get into an argument with the police about what did or didn't happen, so you pled no contest to the domestic assault charges. Now you're here, and the standard protocol for this type of offense is anger management and a few other types of groups.
>
> OFFENDER: Isn't there anything you can do to make it easier?

PROBATION OFFICER: I'd be glad to work with you on that. To do that, we first need something like 6 months of good progress. So it's just a matter of navigating these first 6 months. It depends on you.

OFFENDER: But why do I have to do all these things when I'm not guilty? I know what happened, and it's ridiculous that I'm stuck in here, and that I have to talk about issues I don't have. I went to that anger management orientation class, and it's going to be a waste of my time. But if I don't do it, there's no way I'd be considered for early release.

PROBATION OFFICER: Kind of a rough spot to be in. The choice is yours. Since neither of us has any control over that, what can I do to help you through the process?

The probation officer is not drawn into an argument. By listening and emphasizing the offender's personal responsibility, he or she works with the offender without taking sides on the issue of innocence or guilt. The process of engagement and the spirit of MI remind us that our field has often prized obedience and compliance over behavior change. Using a guiding style in these situations can make a substantial difference in outcomes for our offender clients.

THE DRAMA OF CHANGE

Recognizing and responding to sustain talk and discord is an opportunity to stay within the MI frame and to promote successful change. By arguing for the status quo or expressing discord, the offender is rehearsing a script that has been played out many times before. Whether it's reacting to sustain talk or discord, experiencing dishonesty, or handling violations and dispensing sanctions, there is an expected role for you to play—one that the offender knows well. Your lines are predictable. If you do as others have done, the script will come to the same conclusion as it has before.

But you can rewrite your role. Your part in the play need not be the dry predictable lines that the client expects. In a way, MI is like improvisational theater. No two sessions run exactly the same way. If one actor changes his or her role, the plot heads in a new direction. Tension is often the life of a play. It is the twist that adds drama and excitement to the plot. Viewing sustain talk or discord as a perverse character flaw is a sad mistake, for these lie at the very heart of human change. They arise from the motives and struggles of the actors and foreshadow possibilities in the play's end. Nothing is certain, and with offenders, you'll occasionally find violations and sanctions in the script. The true art of MI is realized in recognizing and handling these tensions. It is on this stage that the drama of change plays to its conclusion.

AUTHORS' NOTE

This chapter is adapted from Walters, Clark, Gingerich, and Meltzer (2007).

CHAPTER 13

THE RISE
OF MOTIVATIONAL
INTERVIEWING

Greatness lies, not in being strong, but in the right using of
strength; and strength is not used rightly when it serves only to
carry a man above his fellows for his own solitary glory.
—HENRY WARD BEECHER

MI is certainly a versatile way of initiating and continuing conversations with people who struggle with ambivalence, with a goal of helping them resolve their ambivalence and make a decision about change.
Thus far in this text we have emphasized what MI is and what makes it
work, as well as when, how, and with whom to use it. Now, however,
we take a step back to examine how this approach—originally applied
within the context of addiction treatment—gained traction in offender
work. As we noted in Chapter 1, several elements of MI have made
it attractive to a range of offender service systems. Rapid diffusion
within these systems followed, though why MI has become so popular
in offender work remains a relevant question. To answer this, we will
discuss a number of related concepts. First, we must examine where
MI came from to better understand its introduction in the world of
offender rehabilitation and reentry. We must also then consider how
MI was initially implemented in offender service agencies and offender
research, as well as how its use with offenders has shaped the practice
of MI. Finally, we will discuss why MI has remained so popular among

those who work with offenders. These topics will then lead into our next chapter, focusing on the implementation and sustainability of MI in offender systems.

WHERE DID MI COME FROM?

MI emerged from the field of addiction treatment in the United States in the 1980s. William Miller coined the term "MI" to describe a way of working with people in which he did not confront or disagree with the client's "resistance" but instead responded in a way that seemed to diminish resistance, primarily through the use of reflective listening (Miller, 1983). He arranged the conversation in such a way that the client made the arguments for change, rather than falling into a pattern in which the therapist pushed for change and the client argued against it. While on sabbatical in Australia in 1989, Miller met Steve Rollnick, who had been expanding this work in the United Kingdom. Together they wrote the first edition of the now-classic text on MI (Miller & Rollnick, 1991).

This initiated a rapid diffusion of MI across multiple helping disciplines—to the point where it is perhaps easier to name the helping fields that have *not* incorporated this approach than to name those that have. Still, a short list of selected areas of focus provides a sense of the expansiveness of this diffusion.

- Family violence (e.g., Kistenmacher & Weiss, 2008; Musser et al., 2008)
- School systems (e.g., Rollnick, Kaplan, & Rutschman, 2016)
- Gambling (e.g., Carlbring, Jonsson, Josephson, & Forsberg, 2010; Diskin & Hodgins, 2009; Petry, Weinstock, Ledgerwood, & Morasco, 2008)
- Dental–oral health (e.g., Carlisle, 2014)
- Dietary changes (e.g., Clifford & Curtis, 2016)
- Diabetes care (e.g., Steinberg & Miller, 2015)
- Pain management (e.g., Frey, 2008; Rau, Ehlebracht-König, & Petermann, 2008)
- Social work (e.g., Hohman, 2012)

MI has been applied with adolescents and adults, people challenged with brain injury or varied mental illnesses, and even to assist mothers with safe water practices in remote African villages (Thevos, Quick, &

Yanjuli, 2000). As one can easily see, the dispersion of MI has reached far and wide.

HOW DID MI BEGIN WITH OFFENDERS?

Though MI began with addictions treatment, a field that naturally intersects with "offender work" given that many persons involved in such treatment have used illegal substances or engaged in illegal behavior as the result of their substance use, the first attempt to use MI with offenders is perhaps impossible to specify. At first glance, some will say it started earlier in Europe than in the United States (with the exception of addictions treatment, as noted above). In the United Kingdom, Mason (personal communication, 2015) reports that there was great interest in the 1980s after the publication of Miller's initial paper (Miller, 1983). By the late 1980s, a 2-day MI workshop was a regular part of the in-service training program for supervising officers who worked for the Birmingham (England) Probation Services (West Midlands). Thus, criminal justice populations have been part of MI research from the beginning, contributing to a continued growing interest following the publication of the first MI text in 1991 (Miller & Rollnick, 1991). The earliest publication cited in the library database Criminal Justice Abstracts under the keyword *motivational interviewing* is from 1999—with subsequent references (2000–2002) involving the use of MI in drug courts. In the next 5 years (1999–2004), there were 68 publications involving offender work that cited the use of MI, including a text describing efforts for motivating offenders to engage in therapy (McMurran, 2002).

While these 68 publications show an early interest in addressing offender motivation, the term "punishment" was cited in 2,045 justice publications during the same 5-year span. However, interest in MI accelerated sharply in 2004, perhaps initiated by the push in U.S. correctional systems for evidence-based practices to reduce offender recidivism. MI gained notice in the field, as it was already established as an evidence-based practice in addictions work. The National Institute of Corrections and the Crime and Justice Institute developed a model for implementing evidence-based practices and improving reentry outcomes for offenders in the community. This culminated in a publication highlighting MI as a practice to enhance intrinsic motivation (Joplin et al., 2004). During the next 10 years, MI was a keyword in 435 offender-related publications—a 600% increase from the previous period.

WHAT BROUGHT ABOUT THIS CHANGE?

In the 1980s, punishment and incarceration were the predominant responses to offender behavior. During this "decade of punishment" (Clear & Frost, 2013) the field used coercive power and authority to guide offender interactions. But rather than helping staff reach their objectives, this demanding and directive style only increased offender resistance. This left offender service personnel overwhelmed by roadblocks that many now realize were self-imposed (Bogue et al., 2004; McMurran, 2002).

During this extended period of punishment in the United States, temporary compliance took center stage while rehabilitation and lasting behavior change were relegated to the background (Clark, 2006). MI appeared as an alternative to this overly directive style, offering tools to influence positive behavior change. But would MI fit? Would offenders respond differently than other people to change interventions? Miller & Rollnick (2013) state:

> One consideration is that, by virtue of being deprived of prior freedoms, a higher than usual level of reactance might be present and an oppositional response could be anticipated to confrontational approaches that further challenge autonomy. Studies have supported a better response to MI than to a more directing style among people with higher reactance levels (Grodin, 2006; Karno & Longabaugh, 2005a, 2005b; Karno, Longabaugh, & Herbeck, 2009). *From this perspective, MI may be a particularly appropriate style in working with offenders.* (p. 344, emphasis added)

As with other helping disciplines, evidence-based practice has been a boon for corrections and other offender systems, though it sometimes breeds cynicism when expensive programs fail to produce desired effects. Designing services based on the risk–needs–responsivity (RNR) model (Andrews et al., 1990; Bonta & Andrews, 2007) has become the predominant practice approach for offender populations (see Chapter 1). Yet though the RNR model has shown positive results in promoting effective reentry and reduced recidivism (e.g., Bonta & Andrews, 2007; Dowden & Andrews, 1999, 2000; Harkins & Beech, 2007), it is neither perfect, nor perfected (e.g., Polaschek, 2012). The most persistent criticism of RNR is that its application seems to assume "one size fits all"; how to include and harness human motivation and individual differences is vague or lacking (Ward & Maruna, 2007). MI, in contrast, offers teachable methods for including individual differences and establishing the working relationship—vital ingredients for positive outcomes (see Chapter 5).

WHAT MAKES THIS APPROACH SO POPULAR IN OFFENDER WORK?

In Chapter 1, we described several considerations for offender agencies interested in adopting MI. These included such things as the evidence base of MI and the desire to be part of behavior change. But there is more. Here, we consider seven reasons that MI has spread so quickly throughout the field of offender work.

1. *There are limits to the coercive approach.* We have written extensively on the limits of a tough and coercive style both within this book and elsewhere (see Chapters 1, 3, & 4; Clark, 2006, 2008). A majority of staff members who work with offenders in community supervision, corrections, and forensic mental health systems understand the limits to a coercive style. As we have noted earlier within this text, coercion does little to strengthen lasting behavior change and may indeed hamper meaningful collaborative partnerships that are necessary to promote successful offender rehabilitation and reentry. Those who work in offender systems are rarely taught how to assess or improve motivation, nor the importance of the processes of human behavior change. After several decades of "confront, challenge, and change" (Barry, 2007), it became obvious that MI better explains why confrontation and challenge in fact lead in the opposite direction from change. The rise of MI in offender systems originates from this realization.

> *Those who work in offender systems are rarely taught how to assess or improve motivation.*

2. *Agents of offender systems want to be more helpful.* Tolle (1999) said, "I cannot tell you anything that deep within you don't already know. You recognize the truth when you hear it" (p. 122). People who choose to work with offenders want to be helpful, and the majority hope their clients will succeed. It may be optimistic to assume that large, bureaucratic agencies, facilities, or offender systems are dissatisfied with the pursuit of compliance but instead seek meaningful change. However,

change remains a shared goal. Change means rehabilitation and effective reentry. Many who work within these systems understand the conventional approach and its implementation, but it does not radically change them or inspire them to greatness in their everyday jobs. In contrast, the transformative approach embraced by MI will not only change clients but also the staff persons using it. In training, many individuals describe how using MI brought them both renewal and transformation. As noted by one trainee returning for an MI booster session, "It's not only what it did for my offenders, but it's what it did for me."

Blame is unnecessary when the goal follows the spirit of MI. Initially, poor outcomes often lead to blaming the "unmotivated" offender. If problems continue, they are blamed on the staff who work with the offenders. Many staff members are merely doing what they have been taught, or what was modeled for them—arguing someone into change when he or she does not want to be changed. Such an approach is ineffective and exhausting and only furthers efforts to find someone to blame rather than examining the root of the problem. The mind-set and heart-set of partnership, acceptance, compassion, and evocation offer a firm foundation for better practice, and ultimately, better helping.

MI offers the tools that allow you to be more helpful. For example, following training in MI, offenders have rated their probation officers as more helpful and understanding, which in turn has promoted more prosocial attitudes toward crime and reoffending (Harper & Hardy, 2000; Hohman, Doran, & Koutsenok, 2009; Spiller & Guelfi, 2007). This is noteworthy in light of what we discussed in Chapter 5—it was the offender's evaluation of the alliance, rather than the officer's, that proved a more accurate predictor of outcomes (Bachelor & Horvath, 1999). MI may thus bring the desire to help closer to reality.

3. *People recognize MI.* In our years of training correctional, community supervision, and forensic mental health staff, we have been approached many times by workshop participants who remarked, "I've been doing this [MI] with offenders, but I just never called it anything" or "It's great to finally put a name to this, because I've been doing this all along." These individuals knew to build a strong connection between themselves and the offender, finding that a certain type of relationship and interactive style was critical to facilitating positive outcomes for offenders (Dowden & Andrews, 2004). Such persons are attracted to the MI approach to understanding resistance (e.g., when you push, they only push back) and avoiding interviewing traps. Still, the belief that "I already do this" is strong when training begins with open-ended questions and reflective listening but wavers somewhat when participants learn the intricacies of focusing and evoking. It's not as simple as it looks at first.

4. MI helps you do your job better. If procedures, methods or approaches are to be attractive and "catch on" with a variety of personnel, such approaches must be, above all else, practical and helpful. Without buy-in from those meant to implement a new strategy, implementation is mere wishful thinking. Yet MI has seemingly accomplished these goals. Many agencies, systems, and organizations devoted to offender rehabilitation and reentry have successfully implemented MI as a core component of their work. This involves several elements: boosting openness and cooperation, broad applicability, easily observed and early success, and compatibility with busy schedules and even competing goals.

First, MI facilitates openness and cooperation. Staff who work with offenders are faced with mountains of paperwork, multiple responsibilities, and seemingly never-ending routine and as-needed requirements. All of these duties rely on the ability to gather accurate information from offenders, hopefully without the awkwardness and discord that often result from working with uncooperative interviewees. However, as we have discussed throughout the early chapters of this text, offenders often have prior experiences, doubts, and expectations that lead them to be understandably uncooperative. Under these conditions, the benefit of using MI becomes evident. People disclose information more freely and accurately when they are being listened to, respected, and supported. Active listening, coupled with MI's ability to reduce client resistance, creates a more genuine and less defensive conversational environment. MI helps influence behavior change, and those who use it quickly see that and help spread the word.

Second, MI can be broadly applied, easily supplementing other tasks. Supervisors, therapists, and line staff may ask: "How can MI assist with all that I have to do?" It would make little sense to limit offender practice to MI, and MI allows for flexibility. Switching back and forth between MI and other styles or strategies—interchanging or initiating approaches depending on the task at hand—is a more realistic option (Longabaugh, Zweben, Locastro, & Miller, 2005; Miller, 2004). Importantly, MI can be useful from beginning to end for any given offender. From our experience as trainers and proponents of MI with offenders, people report that they "never put it down." This approach is applicable for duties ranging from intake and case planning, monitoring, and supervision to case termination or transfer. Still, this practice is not a cure-all; nor is it something just for the good times or favorable situations. Many continue with MI even when sanctions must be used with the client (Chapter 12). When the spirit takes root, the mind-set and heart-set of partnership, acceptance, compassion, and evocation become a firm foundation for offender work.

Third, early results are obvious. Research is clear about the impact of first impressions (Bar, Neta, & Linz, 2006; Yu, Saleem, & Gonzalez, 2014). Verbal and nonverbal cues in the first client meeting not only set the tone for the initial conversation but color the developing relationship. From the first greeting and handshake, relationships can begin collaboratively rather than gearing up for a boxing match. It may take time to adjust to hearing "You're different" or "Nobody has ever talked to me like this." People describe a mixture of shock and joy when tough and unyielding clients respond with cooperation and refreshing openness (Bogue, Diebel, & O'Connor, 2008).

Fourth, MI works with busy schedules. A common complaint among offender agencies is that a high caseload and lack of time interfere with effective practice. Can you do MI in 5 minutes? Well, can you ruin motivation in 5 minutes? *Of course.* You can make a difference in only a few minutes, and you will likely be more effective with this approach than with finger-wagging, threats, or warnings (e.g., Soria, Legido, Escolano, Lopez Yeste, & Montoya, 2006). Likewise, only a few confrontational responses are required to increase client resistance and undermine behavior change (Miller et al., 1993), and only adding MI to confrontation is not enough (e.g., Miller & Mount, 2001). It is just as important to suppress these directive habits as it is to introduce new ones.

5. *Positive outcomes for offenders.* Since 1990, the number of scientific publications on the effectiveness of MI has doubled about every 3 years. There are currently more than 1,300 publications on this approach with offenders. It is recognized as an evidence-based practice for a variety of focus areas. And with regard to recidivism, we know that intervening at the human service level is crucial for effectively addressing the problem of criminality (Bonta et al., 2008). In other words, an approach like this one that emphasizes specific interactions between and offender and a member of an offender services agency has proven successful through decades of research (Bogue et al., 2008), and early evaluations of MI with offender work in New Zealand demonstrate a positive impact on recidivism rates (Anstiss et al., 2011).

6. *Adherence to core correctional practice.* There are five dimensions of effective core correctional practice (CCP) designed to enhance the potential of rehabilitation programs for offenders (Andrews & Kiessling, 1980). One dimension of CCP includes "relationship factors." This is described by Dowden and Andrews (2004) as "the interpersonal influence exerted by the correctional staff member . . . maximized under conditions characterized by open, warm and enthusiastic communication. An equally important consideration is the development of mutual respect and liking between the officer and correctional staff member" (p. 205). The effectiveness of these core relationship skills has been amply supported by correctional and criminal justice researchers (Andrews & Kiessling, 1980; Dowden & Andrews, 2004; Taxman, Cropsey, Melnick, & Perdoni, 2008; Trotter, 1996), most notably producing significant reductions in recidivism (Trotter, 1996). Understandably, MI can produce the environment in which these relationship factors flourish. In fact, the emphasis on mutual respect, warmth, empathy, and openness noted by Dowden and Andrews (2004) is shared by CCP and MI.

Though these principles have been noted specifically within the context of correctional practice, one can easily imagine how the relationship factors noted above are applicable to the broader realm of offender work. Especially noteworthy are research reports about what works with high-risk offenders, again highlighting relationship factors. Robinson, VanBenschoten, Alexander, & Lowenkamp (2011) noted that outcomes were improved when community supervision officers received "additional training in interpersonal communication, particularly an officer's ability to collaborate with the client (rather than being authoritative), connect in an empathic way, and evoke from the client thoughts and feelings regarding behavior" (p. 14). These elements are a profound description of what we find in the spirit of MI. Thus, MI is attractive to supervisors, practitioners, and line staff members in offender environments in that it provides a framework for developing these relationship skills.

A PARADIGM SHIFT

The criminologist Francis T. Cullen has noted, "The punishment paradigm [has] reached the point of exhaustion. We cannot imprison and punish out of the crime problem" (2007, p. 717). Cullen then calls for a need to reaffirm rehabilitation as the guiding force of offender policy and practice and offers five reasons for this change:

1. Rejecting rehabilitation was a mistake.
2. Punishment does not work.
3. Rehabilitation does work.
4. The public likes rehabilitation, even if it is a "liberal" idea.
5. Rehabilitation is the moral thing to do.

Critics of rehabilitation lie in wait, hoping to capitalize on inevitable setbacks as rehabilitation reasserts itself (Cullen, 2007). However, this should not deter us from considering an important paradigm shift. The call for a return to rehabilitation has been frequent and global (Bonta et al., 2008; Burnett & McNeill, 2005; Clear & Frost, 2013; Farrall, 2002; Lewis, 2014; McNeill, 2012; Maruna & Immarigeon, 2004; McMurran, 2002; Ward & Maruna, 2007). These concerns, and their link with the spirit and practice of MI, can be viewed further in Table 13.1 (see also Lowenkamp, Holsinger, Robinson, & Cullen, 2012).

These comparisons highlight only a portion of what MI can offer. The rapid diffusion and level of integration across the world of offender practice implies that MI offers what many criminal justice, correctional, and forensic mental health agencies are seeking in their efforts to establish rehabilitative goals.

However, to say that offender agencies have shifted paradigms from punishment back to rehabilitation is not an automatic endorsement for the use of MI. To that end, Miller and Rollnick (2013, pp. 335–336) offered questions to ask yourself if you are considering the applicability of MI to your work. These questions may be particularly relevant as you consider changes in the view of offender needs we have just discussed:

1. Are there—or should there be—conversations about change happening?
2. Will the outcomes for those you serve be influenced by the extent to which they make changes in their lives or behavior?
3. Is helping or encouraging people to make such changes part of your service—or should it be?
4. Are the people you serve often reluctant or ambivalent about making changes?
5. Is accessing services—along with adherence and retention in your services—a significant concern?
6. Do staff struggle with or complain about people who are "unmotivated," "resistant," or "difficult"?

Miller and Rollnick (2013) posed these questions with the assumption that if agencies responded to each with "yes," it suggests that MI

TABLE 13.1. Offender Practice Concerns and MI

Concerns about current offender service practices (Lowenkamp et al., 2012)	Same concerns, addressed through MI
The evidence-based practice movement is widespread but shallow. It fails to see the person as an individual and separate the offender from his or her illegal behavior.	Viewing the person as bad and undeserving of forgiveness or another chance is incompatible with an MI style. (Chapter 2)
More research is needed regarding the relationship and empathy, and what they should look like. We also lack specifics on how to teach these skills to personnel working with offenders or how to put such skills into practice. Empathy may, in fact, be most important.	In the spirit of MI and acceptance, we listen to offenders in order to understand the world as they see it. Accurate empathy is critical. (Chapter 2)
Many agencies fail to recognize a need for more than one treatment, or for flexible approaches to offender management. This leads to frustration when the one prevailing treatment fails to work.	One can switch flexibly back and forth between MI and other styles as is needed, depending on the task. One can stop MI and similarly start it. (this chapter)
Roles within offender systems are often blurred. Staff must establish trusting and functional relationships with the offenders they work with while still performing their job responsibilities. The two roles must be more fluidly blended.	MI allows you to develop a collaborative relationship in the context of a power difference between you and the offender. This does not, however, call for you to suspend your responsibility for reporting problematic behavior, or the reality that problem behavior may carry sanctions. (Chapter 2)

might be of assistance in their work with clients. In our experience, those who work in offender service agencies not only answer "yes" to these questions, but that even the questions themselves bring a sense of renewed hope and excitement to our field.

Still, things may not be as straightforward as you would like them to be. Even if the responses to such questions are "yes," there may exist attitudes that run counter to the spirit of MI. Imagine dominant assumptions like these:

"The only language these knuckleheads understand is to get in their face and try to put the fear in them so they'll listen to what you're saying."

"I don't have time to put work into people who aren't unmotivated."

"Most of the people I work with don't want to change no matter what I do. The issue is that they don't care."

"I'm the expert here. If these people knew how to change, they wouldn't have ended up on my caseload."

"I don't have time to listen to people and their stories. I've got way too much paperwork."

Even in an environment this closed or authoritarian, we still think one could effectively use MI. Even a small group of staff—or just one person!—who are client-centered can make a difference. For example, even within a very confrontational 21-day residential alcohol treatment program, simply adding a single session of MI after admission doubled abstinence rates after discharge in comparison to treatment as usual (i.e., without the single session of MI; Brown & Miller, 1993). Unaware of whether or not clients had received a session of MI, direct care staff rated the clients who had received the intervention as more motivated, adherent, and having a better prognosis posttreatment. Their impressions were correct.

Even a small group of staff—or just one person!—who are client-centered can make a difference.

This leads us into our next chapter, where we'll continue the systems view with a practical look at implementation science. Now that we have examined how MI may bridge the gap between desired outcomes and real-world practice with offenders, we must examine how it works. How does what we know—and what we do—stack up with the science? What strategies and methods have offender service agencies relied upon as they merge MI into their existing systems? From single-event trainings with only a few interested staff to progressive, whole-system roll-outs, what do we know so far about training, implementation, and sustainability? What should be replicated, and what should be avoided? A rich discussion awaits in the next chapter.

CHAPTER 14

IMPLEMENTATION AND SUSTAINABILITY

Excellence is an art won by training and habituation. We are
what we repeatedly do. Excellence then, is not an act, but a
habit.
—ARISTOTLE

I hated every minute of training, but I said, "Don't quit. Suffer
now and live the rest of your life like a champion."
—MUHAMMAD ALI

We've examined the practice of MI and how it differs from conventional
(typically directive) methods in offender work. We've discussed important learning strategies for using this approach with a variety of offenders in a variety of offender systems. We've also considered reasons why
this approach is so attractive and appealing for offender agencies, examining the benefits it offers for influencing positive behavior change. All
of this leads to an important question: *How do you integrate MI into
your own agency's work with offenders?* In this chapter, we will briefly
provide some initial observations to help set the stage for implementing
and sustaining MI training in your agency. Then we will discuss learning transfer and agency integration practices, concluding with a discussion of differing modalities of training and the use of new technologies
to more effectively and efficiently provide training in large offender service agencies.

AN IMPORTANT INTRODUCTORY NOTE:
THINGS TO DO (AND A FEW THINGS NOT TO)

Before we delve deeply into methods of learning, here are six things we
have learned from over a decade of MI training for offender work that
we hope you will consider as you contemplate integration in your own
agency.

1. *Implementation comes in many sizes.* Whether the agency serves
a country, state/province, region, or community, or urban, metro, or
rural jurisdiction, MI can be successfully implemented across venues. In
small agencies, two or three practitioners may import MI into their personal practice—even without the blessing or oversight of management
(i.e., "We didn't ask—we just did it"). In the United States, multiple state
departments of corrections have implemented MI practices throughout
their institutions, as have the Federal Bureau of Prisons and the Probation and Pretrial Services of the U.S. Courts. This demonstrates the
flexibility and versatility of MI referenced in Chapter 13—MI can be
implemented in small specialized groups or across the full complement
of services with varied offenders, as well as at intake or throughout the
continuum of rehabilitation and community reentry.

2. *MI is more difficult to learn than many think it is.* There is no
minimum or sufficient "dose" of training to guarantee competence in
MI. There is a certain level of training needed to change staff behavior, though another level is needed to change offender behavior. MI
is a skills-based practice, and these skills are very much like learning
how to play golf or fly an airplane. Mastery is more than claiming a
certain number of hours of didactic training. Unfortunately, staff often
overestimate their skill level (Hohman & Matulich, 2010), believing
themselves to be more proficient than they are. Fortunately, some staff
members learn and develop the skills quickly, showing early mastery.
This is not always the case, however, and one must plan for continued
skills training and reinforcement.
People also easily fall prey to the
"inoculation effect," or believing
that after minimal training, they
are in no need of more. Instead,
implementation is a process rather
than an event. For instance, paint-
ing a room in a house is a specific,
one-time event. When it is finished,

> *There is a certain level of training needed to change staff behavior, though another level is needed to change offender behavior.*

you can complete the job and marvel at the new look. In contrast, overall home upkeep is a process—one of monitoring the status of multiple rooms, appliances, and systems, as well as prompt response and repair of emerging problems, routine maintenance, and continual budgeting for anticipated future needs. Such preparation is continual. The same holds true for learning and practicing MI.

3. *MI is not always given its due in traditional offender treatment approaches.* There are many offender treatment programs to choose from—all aimed at reducing recidivism for community safety—and many have received some empirical support. Some of the more well-known models include Effective Practices in Community Supervision (EPICS; University of Cincinnati Correctional Institute), Staff Training Aimed at Reducing Re-arrest (STARR; Robinson et al., 2011), varied cognitive behavioral treatments, and as variations of the cognitive behavioral model, Thinking for a Change (T4C; Bush, Glick, Taymans, & Guevera, 2011) and the Strategic Training Initiative in Community Supervision (STICS; Bonta et al., 2010). These approaches are based on the RNR framework that is part of the larger principles for evidence-based practice in offender work (e.g., Andrews & Carvell, 1998; Bogue et al., 2004; Bonta & Andrews, 2007; Dowden & Andrews, 1999, 2000). Where does MI fit?

When offender treatment programs claim to use MI, there may be little adherence to what we have described so carefully in this text. Our fear is that it is merely a mirage—MI is visible from afar but vanishes upon closer inspection. This is not the fault of these programs or those who train their staff. Instead, this may result when people underestimate the ease with which MI can be disseminated and implemented in a given agency. To us, it makes most sense to begin with engagement, followed by increased cooperation and influencing offender motivation. However, many agencies implement their own programming first, adding a smattering of "MI" as an afterthought, for only those who prove difficult or resistant. This is not nearly as effective as starting with MI to pave the way for more effective treatment later.

4. *Successful preparation and implementation of organizational change occur in a given order.* Research examining implementation science in human service organizations identifies six sequential stages (Fixsen, Naoom, Blase, Friedman, & Wallace, 2005): (a) Exploration and adoption; (b) program installation; (c) initial implementation; (d) full operation; (e) innovation; and (f) sustainability. Unfortunately, our experiences show that many offender service agencies begin in the

middle—training and implementation. Instead, what we should take from this list is what must occur *first*. Gathering information, finding support among staff and management, reassigning agency resources, reorganizing or realigning staff, and modifying policy and procedures— these are critical steps before the first training group is ever assembled. The problem in most offender agencies or systems is that these early efforts are overlooked; implementation begins with training.

Grant funding may drive much of this implementation sequence. Many grants begin with training; funding is provided for initial training, as well as continuing the service or program once training has ended. Funding often neglects the early buy-in stages that are so important for effective and lasting implementation and MI may be dismissed by staff as "the flavor of the month." Agencies would be better served by deliberate attention to organizational readiness. Otherwise, it is a backward scramble to put necessary supports in place once training— and implementation efforts—have already begun. Early and necessary considerations include:

- Interest and buy-in from staff
- Interest and buy-in from management
- Clear articulation of why MI is needed, who will use it, how it will be used, and who must be trained
- How the program or agency intends to sustain MI (e.g., continued training, coaching, and feedback)
- How management or administration will be involved in sustainability
- Planned reallocation of responsibility for in-house trainers and coaches to allow for additional job tasks
- The role of MI programming in job evaluations, job responsibilities, and hiring practices
- Mechanisms for evaluating adherence to MI practice for programs and individual personnel

Some additional guidance has been provided by Dickinson, Edmundson & Tomlin (2006), who found that agencies had more success with implementing MI if they developed clear aims (e.g., increase client retention, reduce client resistance, and increase treatment success), articulated plans for development and implementation, had sufficient internal funding, and obtained commitment from senior leadership.

5. *The extinction effect must be considered.* Although known by many names—diminished skills, practice drift, competence drain, or skill erosion—the extinction effect is a very real problem in implementation of MI (Baer et al., 2004; Bogue, Pampel, & Pasini-Hill, 2013; Dickinson et al., 2006). Learned skills can diminish over time, and people will also change important components of their practice, either replacing learned methods with preferred variations, or simply forgetting or disregarding important elements of the practice.

Consider what it takes to learn to play the piano. One or two days of intensive and all-day instruction, possibly followed by additional training and practice over the course of several more days, and you would have a rudimentary working knowledge of the piano, as well as ability to play a few basic pieces. But what if you didn't play again for months, or a year? And what if you have no further lessons? The consequences are obvious—you would no longer remember how to play, and you would be unlikely to initiate the effort. This is a common occurrence with MI and other approaches in offender settings. The lack of posttraining follow-up causes even skilled and well-intentioned staff members to forget what they have previously learned, and they are unlikely to use these skills in the future. Later in this chapter we will examine what works to combat the extinction effect.

6. *New learning requires coaching and feedback.* Feedback is fundamental for any kind of learning, and immediate feedback that occurs in the moment is even more helpful. Does your agency provide ongoing coaching and feedback after training concludes? If the norm in your agency is to provide only the training, then you're in the majority. Whether training involves singular or multiple sessions, most agencies end their implementation effort with training, neglecting the importance of ongoing coaching and feedback to enhance learning and practice. Staff build skills with greater speed and competency under the helpful eye of a coach who offers feedback and correction.

> *Does your agency provide ongoing coaching and feedback after training concludes?*

LEARNING TRANSFER
AND AGENCY INTEGRATION

What does it take to learn MI? Above, we have listed several important things to take into consideration to more effectively implement MI within your agency or system. When it comes to the practicalities of implementation, several additional topics are relevant.

Workshop Training

A 1- or 2-day workshop will certainly expose the participant to the concepts of MI and should include some experiential practice. A 2-day follow-up (advanced) training allows for further exercise and skills practice. To reach expertise (full competency), one would need continued coaching and feedback. A competent workshop series should include a wide-ranging menu of MI concepts. MI, as applied in offender work, is not a single technique but rather a combined set of interviewing skills. There are specific learning tasks associated with the core skills of this approach (Miller & Moyers, 2006; Miller & Rollnick, 2013):

- Understanding the spirit of MI (PACE; Chapter 2)
- Developing skill and comfort with reflective listening (Chapter 3) and OARS skills (Chapter 6)
- Identifying important change goals (Chapter 8)
- Exchanging information and providing advice using an MI style (Chapter 6)
- Recognizing change talk and sustain talk (Chapter 9)
- Evoking change talk (Chapter 10)
- Responding to change talk in a way that strengthens it (Chapter 10)
- Responding to sustain talk and discord in a way that does not amplify it (Chapters 10 and 12)
- Developing hope and confidence (Chapter 10)
- Timing and negotiating a change plan (Chapter 11)
- Strengthening commitment (Chapter 11)
- Flexibly integrating MI with other skills and practices (Chapter 13)

There is no exact sequence to these topics, and they may not always be learned in order. Some trainees may already possess a few of these skills. But for others, these topics are completely new, and the learner must start from the beginning. Some topics or tasks like reflective listening are foundational to the practice of MI and must be learned before more advanced skills, like deepening change talk, are attempted. What is clear is that learning all of these tasks—and competently using them—is simply not feasible during only 2 days of training.

What an agency can expect from an introductory MI workshop is to gain some knowledge of the approach. A 2-day introductory training can acquaint the trainee with the purpose, spirit, and core concepts of

MI. At a basic level, the goal is for people to decide if they want to continue learning and using this in their work with offenders. Continuing with an advanced session of 2 more days is helpful to adequately introduce these foundational skills and provide some time for practice. Current research (Hartzler & Espinosa, 2011; Forsberg, Ernst, & Farbring, 2011) has found benefit for criminal justice personnel who go beyond the introductory 2-day workshop to complete an advanced session. Agencies have also accessed telephone or web-based training to continue learning after initial on-site sessions have ended. These blended learning formats (face-to-face with phone conferencing or computer-based training) will be discussed in the next section.

In summary, varied levels of training, coaching and feedback, or providing a menu of options including these elements can be helpful in effectively learning and using MI. An introductory session will serve to explain the practice, raise interest, and begin initial skills building. Advanced training can produce changes in staff behavior. We have also known "prodigies" who can adopt MI skills after an initial workshop, showing posttraining skill at competence levels. But for the majority, several sessions of training, followed by ongoing feedback and coaching are warranted to produce noticeable changes in client behavior (Miller & Mount, 2001).

Supervision

Most supervisors can relate to feeling overwhelmed and lacking necessary resources. They may be faced with managing too many initiatives at once, with varying goals, constituents, and responsibilities associated with each of these. There is perhaps no perfect ideal for what a supervisor must do in implementing MI for his or her team. In some organizations, the supervisor functions as the primary coach and evaluator for MI, while in other organizations the supervisor insures consistency and continuity of practice, making sure the MI coach has what is needed.

Ideally, supervisors would receive MI training with follow-up evaluation and coaching of their own. Further, the supervisor would submit tapes of live interview sessions and have them coded by a trained evaluator. Since few supervisors continue to work with clients, they may need to "borrow" a client from someone else. Supervisors would continue this process until they reach a beginning competency level. Training in how to model and supervise staff in MI, as well as learning implementation science, would follow. A supervisor would then possess the skills needed to evaluate his or her staff's proficiency in MI, and would possess the essentials needed to make MI the foundation of his or her agency's practices.

A list of questions from over 100 correctional and criminal justice training seminars (Gingerich, personal communication, August 20, 2015) included "What are the most important behaviors or attributes of effective supervision?" Over 90% of respondents indicated one or both of these: (1) modeling integrity—talk matches walk; and (2) modeling what is expected of staff. In other words, organizational readiness involves staff and supervisors alike. Staff look to supervisors to embrace and model MI's style of communication and extend the spirit of the approach in their supervisory work.

Model implementation plans do not always fit real-world situations. For example, the administrative office that oversees federal probation districts intended for supervisors to provide coaching to staff learning MI, but found that they were unequipped to do so. Instead, they changed tactics and provided funding for districts to find those already qualified to provide such coaching (Alexander, VanBenschoten, & Walters, 2008). This experience likely resonates with supervisors reading this text. Many may self-assess their MI skills as lacking, thus feeling unprepared to provide such training, direction, and feedback themselves (Dickinson et al., 2006).

Agencies help the process by devising strategies that include management and supervision in modeling, coaching, fidelity checks, and implementation plans. Supervisors need not be experts in MI, but they should know enough to know (1) when to help staff, and (2) how to help staff. Understanding implementation science and participating in MI training themselves can prepare supervisors and managers for these responsibilities.

Coaching and Feedback

Many who work with offenders operate in relative isolation, with few people observing their interactions with offenders. Yet learning is impaired in the absence of feedback (e.g., Miller, Yahne, Moyers, Martinez, & Pirritano, 2004), and building a mechanism for staff to receive feedback as they learn enhances performance. Review of your work in session or via audio- or videotapes will offer a large return of investment for the effort. Coaching allows comments, review, reactions, advice, and tips, all of which lead to improvement in your performance. And additionally, the coach should have more experience and skill in MI than the person he or she is instructing.

But what about experienced practitioners? One might think that they need little coaching. However, coaching and feedback may be more important than accumulated experience. A consistent finding in counseling research, for example, is that counselors with many years of practice have no better client outcomes, on average, than those who were only recently trained. This includes findings of little difference between professionals and paraprofessionals, or therapists with varying levels of experience (Christensen & Jacobson, 1994). Similarly, Strupp and Hadley (1979) found that experienced therapists were no more helpful than a group of untrained college professors, while Jacobson and Gurman (1995) noted that novice graduate students may be more effective at couple therapy than trained professionals.

How can this be? Finding no or only small differences in effectiveness between novice and experienced professionals is both surprising and distressing. In contrast, Miller and Rollnick (2013) remind us that one of the most replicated findings in medicine is the effect of experience. A surgeon who has done a particular procedure 2,000 times is simply better at it than someone who has done it twice—the experienced surgeon produces better outcomes, fewer complications, and less adverse effects. How does this fit with counseling research suggesting that experience does not matter? The surgeons get constant feedback. They rarely practice alone, and when there are complications or adverse outcomes, they receive rapid feedback and the guided opportunity to make corrections.

Such coaching and feedback may come from multiple sources. Both trained supervisors and outside experts can perform this role. Later in this chapter we will also discuss the emerging use of in-house trainers, peer coaches, "MI champions," coaching within communities of practice, and web-based training to facilitate peer feedback.

Finally, we sympathize with correctional management teams who find the requirements of effective integration daunting. While it may seem difficult enough to disrupt agency operations to convene multiple training sessions, only to face the further call to provide coaching and feedback, there is no need for despair on this count. Even a modest amount of expert coaching can significantly improve proficiency in MI (Miller & Rollnick, 2004). This may involve as few as five or six individual coaching sessions conducted by telephone for 30 minutes each (Miller & Rollnick, 2004). Your organization can be creative in providing coaching and feedback without further straining already stretched resources, and it goes a great distance toward improving the practice of MI in any setting.

Coding and Fidelity Checks

Despite good training, engaged supervisors, and knowledgeable coaching, you may still face the question of whether or not staff are using MI in their interactions with offenders, and staff may wonder if the coach's feedback is consistent with what others who observe the same session would say. Documenting fidelity to the approach with objective measures can help you answer such questions. Importantly, coding and fidelity checks can answer the following questions:

- Are your staff actually delivering MI?
- To what extent, and of what quality?
- How do staff compare with one another within the agency, and to those outside the agency who also use MI in their work?
- Can you assure outside funding resources or oversight agencies of your adherence to evidence-based practice?

There are several choices currently available to assist in coding sessions and examining fidelity in practice. They differ primarily with regard to what they keep track of during a session. The MI Treatment Integrity (MITI—Version 4.2; Moyers, Rowell, Manuel, Ernst, & Houck, 2016) tracks the interviewer's responses from the coding or scoring of audio recordings of live sessions. This instrument grades the quality and quantity of responses to determine fidelity. The Client Language EAsy Rating (CLEAR; Glynn & Moyers, 2012) Coding System tracks only the client's responses from coding of audio recordings of live sessions. The MI Skills Code (MISC; Moyers, Martin, Catley, Harris, & Ahluwalia, 2003) is a more complex system that is used primarily in clinical research. It assesses both client and staff responses from the coding of audio recordings of live sessions. The Video Assessment of Simulated Encounters-Revised (VASE-R; Rosengren, Hartzler, Baer, Wells, & Dunn, 2008) involves staff watching videotaped client vignettes and then generating written responses to the vignettes that are consistent with specific principles of MI.

A more complete inventory of MI fidelity assessment tools can be accessed at *www.motivationalinterviewing.org/library*. While each has advantages and disadvantages, the MITI and the VASE-R are the two coding schemas most widely used in the field of corrections at the present time. And while it is helpful to use some of the methodologies already available for assessing practice, there is also merit to recording your own sessions with an offender and simply listening to them and taking notes.

Besides listening to the flow of your conversation, Miller and Rollnick (2013) suggest structured tasks that can help you focus on the process of MI rather than the content of the client story. These include:

1. Count your reflections. MI teaches you to first try to understand the offender's story and worldview. Reflections are an active and effective way to understand the person.
2. Count your questions. Are they open, or closed? Open questions encourage the offender to talk so you are better prepared to influence subsequent conversation.
3. Count both reflections and questions. What is your ratio of reflections to questions? A learning goal is to operate with a 2:1 ratio—two reflections for every question.
4. Listen for change talk and sustain talk, keeping count of each. If you're hearing a lot of sustain talk—or more sustain talk than change talk—it may indicate that you're pushing too hard for change.
5. Following the offender's change talk, what did you say next? Advanced trainings in MI emphasize the importance of identifying, responding to, reinforcing, and strengthening change talk.
6. Listen for responses that are inconsistent with an MI style. Only a relatively few directive or confrontational responses can increase client resistance and undermine behavior change. Consistent awareness of this, particularly early in the learning process, can help you stay with the spirit and practice of MI.

You don't have to attend to all of these tasks. Expert coaches know to sort through the individual strengths and challenges of those with whom they work. Such a practice is helpful for self-evaluation as well—select one or two areas of focus for learning and emphasize those as you listen to your own sessions. Set related learning goals, such as increasing your own ratio of reflections to questions, or listening intently for how you respond to change talk. This will also strengthen your ability to teach others and provide them feedback as well.

Sustainability

Adherence to implementation science by offender service agencies is certainly varied. In many organizations and systems, the practice has been to convene large groups for initial training in MI, only to neglect the importance of continued learning. This results in "waves" of training—MI is taught, albeit quickly, to an eager and interested audience, excitement and skills ability fade over time, and several years later, administrators realize that the practice of MI has not taken root within the organization. Renewed efforts follow, but if they follow the same course, the results are the same.

How has this happened? Large, bureaucratic systems are difficult to mobilize. Trainers do not always focus on sustainability as much as they need to. How to import MI into offender systems and maintain it has been an area of intense scrutiny over the past decade (e.g., Alexander, Lowenkamp, & Robinson, 2013; Hartzler & Espinosa, 2011; Hohman et al., 2009). We have already addressed several important aspects of this integration (e.g., workshop training, supervision, coaching and feedback, fidelity checks), and we will now examine several more, including train-the-trainer models, communities of practice, and blended learning. These practices will bolster sustainability of MI within a system and encourage it to thrive.

TRAIN-THE-TRAINER MODELS

Introductory workshop training familiarizes participants with the basics of the spirit and applicability of MI. Advanced sessions foster skill building and competent practice. However, it is difficult to predict how much additional training and coaching are required for any given staff member to reach proficiency. And further, turnover rates in many agencies are high, necessitating continued training for incoming personnel. In-house expertise and support are thus invaluable. Many organizations choose to empower staff within their own ranks to serve as trainers for MI.

Some suggestions for implementing a train-the-trainer initiative are provided in Box 14.1.

Selecting the best candidates for trainers involves the philosophy of "best in = best out." Think beyond traditional roles (i.e., most senior personnel, those with prior counseling experience, personnel in the staff development office) and base your selections on those with the natural skills called for by MI. You may have an implicit feel for those with more natural abilities to engage offenders with an MI style. Here are some additional selection criteria to consider:

- Those who relate best with the offenders in your agency. These are the staff members who excel at establishing helping relationships.

**BOX 14.1. HOW TO TRAIN THE TRAINER:
A "BAKER'S DOZEN" SUGGESTIONS**

---

1. You might want to use an outside consultant or professional (e.g., MINT) trainer. Check references—you want an individual who has facilitated train-the-trainer initiatives for other jurisdictions, preferably involving offender systems.

2. Meet with management and supervisors who have been coached in how to identify staff with skills consistent with MI. Refer managers and supervisors to this chapter for suggestions.

3. Select staff who will participate in the train-the-trainer initiative.

4. Provide 2 days of training in the fundamentals of MI. Though these staff might have had prior (though not recent) training, this may be considered a booster session.

5. A break will allow for observed practice with a supervisor before returning to the worksite.

6. Return for 2 more days of advanced MI training.

7. Submit audio- or videotapes of live sessions to the training consultant for coding and fidelity checks. Sessions are coded for specific competencies in MI, and results are returned with telephone or video-conferenced coaching. The staff person is allowed to enter the train-the-trainer initiative when competency scores are achieved.

8. Trainer candidates are selected based on coding and fidelity results. This may also include provisional candidates, as some may be "just ready" for inclusion at near-competency levels and can quickly reach competency through additional guided practice.

9. Assign homework to candidates who are ready for the train-the-trainer sessions. Candidates should prepare their own modules to present in upcoming sessions.

10. Hold a train-the-trainer session of 2 to 3 days in length, with the new trainers presenting materials to a live audience (e.g., small mock audience) and receiving evaluation and feedback from the expert consultant. Once all training modules have been completed, evaluated, and revised, continue by discussing training strategies and curriculum development, accessing MI

(continued)

BOX 14.1. (*continued*)

---

resources, and considering implementation and sustainability strategies for your agency.

11. Once a train-the-trainer candidate has achieved competency in his or her practice and has completed supervised training, he or she can be awarded a trainer certificate for your particular agency or organization. (Such a certification is agency specific and does not speak to as person's ability to provide training in other settings.)

12. Empower trainers to determine future implementation efforts within the agency or organization. This is facilitated by the outside expert consultant. This group will make recommendations to agency management, though recognizing that all suggestions may not be implemented.

13. Optional coding and coaching training, lasting 3 days or more, may be useful for trainers. This will improve their competency levels in practicing and training MI.

New and practiced personnel are equally likely candidates—this is about innate skill rather than longevity.

- Those with innate talents for empathic regard and a collaborative demeanor.
- Those who are above average in their use of reflective listening skills.
- Those who use many open-ended questions and work to fully understand the problem from the offender's perspective before moving forward.
- Those who are admired and respected by their colleagues.
- Those who voluntarily express interest in the initiative.
- Those who are likely to stay with your agency, as you want to invest your resources wisely.
- Those who demonstrate certain skills necessary to be a good trainer. These include an outgoing personality, high energy level, and the desire to lead others and take initiative to drive agency change.

Importantly, don't restrict yourself to those who self-select for the project. While many may express interest, not all will possess the qualities described above. An informed committee or group of supervisors should play a considerable role in the selection process. Also remember, however, that you need both coaches and trainers. While they have similar skill levels, the difference is their comfort level regarding methods of teaching. Trainers have the outgoing personality and enjoy instructing before an assembled class. Coaches may express hesitation about leading large groups yet feel very comfortable working with small groups in a more intimate setting, providing feedback to keep the effort going outside of the classroom. There are many who express interest in serving as both trainer and coach.

The initial identification, selection, and training of training and coaching personnel are only a beginning. It is all too easy for these initiatives to lose focus, particularly in large agencies. Clarity about the long-term expectations for trainers and coaches will establish from the outset that this involves continuous effort. This will allow you to avoid confusion and most effectively allocate your available resources.

COMMUNITIES OF PRACTICE

Many agencies that have most effectively implemented a sustained effort in MI have relied on peer groups who regularly meet for skills building. While the names of these groups may differ—the brown-bag lunch group, lunch-and-learn, or the Tuesday hour—they share the commonality of peer-supported learning. Learning together with peers can be more enjoyable and effective than learning alone, and meeting regularly with others who share the same interest and passion for improvement can help MI skill development really take off. Not only do group members talk about MI, but they practice skills and trade ideas within a supportive learning community. Take a look at Box 14.2 for some suggestions from people who belong to these communities of practice.

This list of ideas from persons who have participated in communities of practice conveys their commitment to peer learning but also highlights the importance of the environment in facilitating implementation and sustainability of MI programs. From administration to the front line, everyone assumes some ownership and responsibility for adopting an MI style throughout the organization.

Supervisors play an important role in generating and supporting a cohesive, working peer skills group. As a supervisor, you can help form a community of practice groups, help them to secure activities and exercises, provide some expert oversight and coaching, and then shield them

---

**BOX 14.2. SUGGESTIONS FOR IMPLEMENTING
YOUR OWN COMMUNITY OF PRACTICE**

1. Keep it to an hour or less. We love to meet but we're busy.

2. Meet on a consistent day and time. It helps us with our scheduling.

3. Group numbers need to stay small and manageable.

4. Try to keep group members the same. We need to bond and trust each other. We don't do as well with rotating group membership, with members cycling in and out.

5. Community does not always mean harmony. Don't include people who don't want to participate, or who don't want to learn MI.

6. Having an available coach or trainer is very helpful. Otherwise, give us process ideas to use in our group hour (e.g., exercises, discussion topics, sample dialogues between staff member and offender, transcripts of sample MI exchanges, short MI videos to watch, quick check-in tests to take and discuss, written sample dialogue where we have to write in what we would say next). Also useful are self-evaluations we can complete after client interviews or the ability to audio-record ourselves with clients to share with each other.

7. If we can't always have a coach or trainer in the group, allow an expert to sit in periodically, either by phone or in person.

8. We're okay with a supervisor joining us but need to be able to make mistakes in our learning without it influencing our job performance evaluations.

---

from distractions or other responsibilities that may compromise their continuity. In this case, supervisors don't necessarily have to practice MI with clients but can help it survive and support their staff.

BLENDED LEARNING OPTIONS

Initial instruction and training in MI should be followed by continued practice with feedback and coaching to improve and increase skills and to maintain them over time. Our final section examines blended learning options to achieve these goals. "Blended learning" broadly describes the practice of using in-person classroom instruction in combination with distance education via web-based instruction (Bonk & Graham, 2006). In the past, distance education would have meant little more than occasional phone conferencing with small groups or occasional phone coaching and consultation. As technology advanced, offender agencies and other organizations were able to provide training and coaching via not only speakerphone and teleconferencing technology but also web-based instruction, webinars, webcam meetings, video conferencing, and smartphone technology. Can holographic projection be far away?

Offender agencies are populated by enthusiasts who embrace technology, those who are cautious or lukewarm, and those who shun technological change. Gasser and Palfrey (2008) classify technological adaptation by age group: (1) digital natives, those 35 years of age or younger who have largely been raised with current technology or the immediate predecessors of current technological standards; (2) digital settlers, or persons ranging from 40 years or older to retirement age who embraced and learned new technologies as they were able; and (3) digital immigrants, or those 40 years or older to retirement age who feel lost and foreign in the face of new technology. Digital natives represent a sizable portion of staff who work with offenders. They are largely unfamiliar with life without digital networked technology. At the other end of the continuum are those personnel in offender systems who avoid or only begrudgingly and superficially accept minimal technological advancement. The range of technological adaptation in your own agency thus impacts openness and ability to use blended learning techniques.

Of greatest concern is when upper administration or management is comprised of these so-called digital immigrants who are suspicious of new technology or reluctant to employ it. Digital tools are now deeply ingrained in our culture, and more than 12 million web meetings occur every day (Turmel, 2011). These and other technological resources offer helpful options to continue with MI skills building and practice, enhancing its sustainability in a variety of offender service agencies. Blended learning offers several cost-effective options, with those options increasing following the introduction of newer technologies every year. We will now examine several that are gaining greater acceptance as implementation, practice, and sustainability tools for offender agencies and systems.

228   MOTIVATIONAL INTERVIEWING WITH OFFENDERS

Teleconferencing

Though the telephone conference is likely familiar to most readers, there are new developments with this approach that make it attractive to coaches and trainers of MI. Among these are trainings in "pods." In a pod, three staff members are matched with one coach or trainer who leads each session using a speakerphone (i.e., the three staff members are onsite together with the coach/trainer remotely participating) or a multiline call that links individuals from different locations. One pod member may be designated an onsite facilitator to ensure that meetings are organized on a regular basis (e.g., every 2 to 4 weeks) and to coordinate technology and paperwork. Prior to the first session, surveys and a coaching needs analysis may be completed and returned to the pod coach/trainer. Coaching sessions conclude with assignments and tasks given to staff for completion prior to the next meeting.

As with most blended options, the MI coach/trainer or consultant can be obtained from outside the agency, or if the organization has empowered in-house trainers and coaches, the pod may include all internal staff from the same agency, though perhaps different locations within that agency. Many offender agencies span large geographical distances, and this blended learning option can overcome isolation to more easily allow training, coaching, and continued practice to occur.

Videoconferencing

Teleconferencing and videoconferencing both allow for questions, interactions, and role plays, along with observation and feedback. Teleconferencing requires only a telephone with speakerphone or conferencing technology, whereas videoconferencing requires a video camera, microphone, and television monitor—all of which require greater financial and technological resources. However, video cameras can capture facial expressions, gestures, and eye contact, adding another dimension to distance-based learning and practice. Visual images can more easily facilitate role plays, and will also allow for nonverbal cues and behaviors to be incorporated into the practice and coaching of MI skills.

Web Conferencing

Online or web-based meetings add computers to the use of telephones, video cameras, and web cameras for blended learning. There are several options for free or fee-based subscription services in use by many organizations (e.g., WebEx, Go-To-Meeting, Skype), some of which protect and encrypt conversations and transmissions. Web-conferencing options allow an MI trainer or coach to meet with any number of learners in a real-time, collaborative format.

Within many web-conferencing software platforms are options to share computer screens alongside video and audio display, allowing a consultant or trainer to share presentation slides or other files with learners while still interacting onscreen via video and online chat features. Another available option in some platforms is the ability to archive web-conferencing sessions for future reference and viewing, which allows an agency to build a library of recordings for others to view.

Web Courses and Webinars

When used efficiently, classroom training and web courses can parallel and complement one another. Web courses or webinars can be provided before or after scheduled classroom training, either preparing learners in advance or making continued learning more readily accessible. Web courses are offered in varying lengths—usually 45 to 60 minutes—and are commonly presented in a series. Many MI web courses are sequential and require learners to successfully pass an exam at the end of the session before being able to access the next course and thus continue the series. Yet these courses can be forgiving by allowing unlimited access, enabling staff to retake any course at any time so that completing a series is simply a matter of application and diligence. Courses are not shared among learners, but rather access is gained by password and entry codes so only the student of record can access his or her own account. Agency management may also have access so that they may check on the progress of any individual or group.

While first-generation web courses were general text-based slides and true–false or multiple-choice exams with little interaction, engagement, or feedback, newer software has allowed for the development of second-generation web-based courses that allow for constant interaction and corrective feedback. Learners not only complete an exam or other assessment but are told why their answers were right or wrong, with additional explanations to further improved learning transfer. Additionally, with new technologies for web learning, participants are seldom passive. Learners may be called upon to decide, answer, interact, or compose responses, attending to the screen and doing something active on each new screen that appears. Selecting and choosing between clips of MI dialogue, matching planks, decision trees, fill-in-the-blank prompts, "rate that MI response" tasks, and drag-and-drops are all new-generation media interactions that keep the learner active and focused.

Web courses do a wonderful job of learning transfer, but they cannot build skills. In addition to web-based learning modalities, the use of communities of practice can reinforce and apply continued skills learning. These small groups can even run in tandem with web-based content learning.

USE OF NEW TECHNOLOGIES
FOR IMPLEMENTATION AND SUSTAINABILITY

Some management teams easily embrace technology and blended learning options, while others only seem to trust on-site classroom training (e.g., Bozarth, 2010). Single episodes of classroom training by outside providers cannot be sustained over time to provide the ongoing coaching and feedback that is necessary to build skills and sustain an MI program initiative.

Empirical comparisons of classroom and distance learning often find that both modalities enjoy similar rates of learning, and both can be equally motivating (e.g., Bernard et al., 2004; Clark, Bewley, & O'Neil, 2006). While some research shows benefits of distance-learning technology over classroom instruction, and other findings reflect better performance with classroom learning, such discrepancies are often due to differences in instructional design rather than the medium in which information is conveyed (Clark, 1994, 1999; Clark & Mayer, 2007; Mayer, 2005). Anyone can readily recall a session of training that was painful, boring, or held little value. The same can be said for blended learning and distance education. One negative experience is not always reflective of all learning experiences in that modality.

It's a new technological age for offender systems. The same technologies that allow for more effective tracking and management of offenders can also facilitate implementation and sustainability of MI initiatives. Progressive implementation teams understand that a few training sessions alone will not result in competent MI practice. Creative learning approaches, a continued focus on practice and feedback, and consideration of valuable characteristics of trainers and learners can refresh learning efforts and make MI a lasting approach in your organization.

CHAPTER 15

CONSIDERATIONS, CAUTIONS, AND COMMENTS

Strategy is about making choices, trade-offs—it's about deliberately choosing to be different.
—MICHAEL PORTER

You cannot serve from an empty vessel.
—ELEANOR BROWN

The story of MI's evolution in offender rehabilitation and reentry reflects an impressive interplay between research and practice, emphasizing positive and lasting behavior change. This focus on behavior change is helped, in part, by the waning of an era of punishment-oriented strategies and the interest in new approaches for rehabilitation. Included also in this progress are judges, wardens, agency directors, and service providers who want to change their organizational practices.

IMPLEMENTING MI IN THE FACE OF PERCEIVED OBSTACLES: CONSIDERATIONS FOR INFORMED PRACTICE

As we have noted in Chapter 14, the field has substantially advanced in its attention to implementation and sustainability of MI in offender agencies since its initial inception in the 1980s. This was evidenced during the 2010 MINT Forum, when Dean Fixsen, a prominent expert in implementation science, delivered a keynote address describing the stages of implementation (Fixsen & Blasé, 2007; Fixsen, Blase, Horner,

& Sugai, 2009). As noted in Chapter 14, these include (1) exploration, (2) installation, (3) initial implementation, (4) full implementation, (5) innovation, and (6) sustainability. In particular, Fixsen et al. (2009) noted that initial implementation (stage 3) could also be termed the "awkward stage," when there is much ambivalence about starting a new initiative—the status quo is attractive and easy, while moving forward and bringing about change are recognized needs. It is then that communities of practice, administrative support, and other sustainability measures must begin to take root.

But what happens at this important point? In this text, we have described the spirit of MI and why it is so important for offender service organizations. We have reviewed and discussed important foundational aspects of listening and interviewing skills, as well as the core elements of engaging, focusing, evoking, and planning. We additionally noted the proliferation of interest in MI with offenders and the importance of implementation and sustainability efforts within offender systems. This "awkward stage" of initial implementation is the "do or die" point for many offender service agencies. Those who want MI begin to push for it, only to be met with complaints and criticism from those who prefer to maintain the systemic status quo.

Those who push back, complain, and criticize may be a "tough" crowd with abrasive and confrontational styles who champion very specific ideologies about offenders and offender rehabilitation. When asked why these groups so loudly complain, administrators may note that few people like change, or that it's hard to accept that what one has been doing all along may be less effective, ineffective, or even harmful. One must become vulnerable to learn new skills, whereas others attribute their hesitation to an overreliance on the "muscle" approach to offender work or "groupthink" (Janis, 1972).* But perhaps more importantly, why is such a small group of detractors given such due? One manager (to remain anonymous) said it best: "To say nothing made it worse. We realized we needed to offer alternative ideas or to voice our beliefs of what MI and motivational research had taught us. We didn't argue—MI taught us not to do that—but we found we had to offer our opinion. Having a response, without going after them, seemed to quiet the nay-sayers." We learn how to do MI

---

*Groupthink is a psychological phenomenon that occurs within a group of people, in which the desire to perpetuate shared group values results in irrational or dysfunctional decision making. Group members try to minimize conflict and reach a consensus decision without critical evaluation of alternative viewpoints, by actively suppressing dissenting viewpoints, and by isolating themselves from outside influences.

from our clients (Miller & Rollnick, 2013). In practicing MI and keeping with the spirit of the approach, we learn how to best implement MI in offender service systems.

Of greatest help to those facing detractors and continuing questions about the applicability of MI is to address common concerns often expressed by the reluctant minority or administrators who balk at systemwide change initiatives. We will describe and respond to seven of these in this final chapter. For each, we'll include:

- Perceived obstacles (e.g., beliefs, objections to MI)
- How the concern is expressed (e.g., complaints, fears)
- Factors to consider (e.g., values or principles associated with the complaints, your own reactions, and potential responses to the obstacles)

PERCEIVED OBSTACLE 1: MI excuses and collaborates with an offender's denial.

Those who believe MI excuses an offender's denial are focused on uncovering the "truth" in their interactions with offenders. For them, the "truth" is what they already know from police reports or other official sources. It discounts the importance of PACE, described in Chapter 2. The "expert trap" maintains that MI only excuses or rewards an offender's denial of the problem. In expressing this obstacle, you may hear statements like:

"I'm not supposed to be their friend."
"It's important to break down denial rather than just going along with it."
"Offenders just play games and try to con you if you don't confront them."
"I'm not helping them if I just buy into the game."

However, there are important factors to consider:

1. Direct confrontation has little relationship with actual behavior change. In most instances, it damages the relationship and leaves you less able to assist with behavior change.

2. Festervan's (2000) *Survival Guide for New Probation Officers* notes, "Probationers are not your friends. They do not come to 'visit'

with you because they like or admire you. Probationers are criminals" (p. 69). Festervan further states, "Establish a policy for yourself about whether you will offer a handshake to your probationers. Some officers are uncomfortable about this altogether or just with certain probationers. If you are one of these, make it your personal policy never to offer your hand to any client" (p. 104). However, the quality of interpersonal relationships with others, including service providers and supervisory agents, is associated with significant reductions in offending (Dowden & Andrews, 2004) and willingness to consider prosocial alternatives. Developing a collaborative partnership through MI can reduce recidivism, and traditional methods of relating with offenders fail to acknowledge findings from the science of rehabilitation.

3. Direct confrontation—or the righting reflex—only encourages offenders to argue for the problem behavior rather than to move closer to change. Gladwell (2013) posits that the rationale for harsh punishment and the righting reflex is based on flawed conclusions. It is not a mere mathematical equation, in which x (failure to follow sanctions) results in y (increased sanctions). Pain and punishment do not cancel out misbehavior. Traditional punitive assumptions ignore the "principle of legitimacy": "When people in authority want the rest of us to behave, it matters—first and foremost—how *they* behave" (Gladwell, 2013, p. 207).

> When people in authority want the rest of us to behave, it matters—first and foremost—how they behave.

4. Even with a radically different approach like MI, the goal is still the same—to affect meaningful behavior change. We all share the same goals. We must recognize that there are different means through which to achieve them. The question is which approach is more likely to result in change.

PERCEIVED OBSTACLE 2: MI gives the offender a choice about whether or not to follow the rules of the court, which weakens the court's authority.

With an emphasis on autonomy and exploring ambivalence, some may reason that MI allows *too much* choice. Such a view mistakenly assumes that reinforcing the authority of the court or the criminal justice system over allowing for choice results in the offender's automatic acceptance of a need for change. You may hear this belief expressed in several ways:

"Community supervision is a privilege that offenders need to earn. They have to accept what they've done wrong in order to earn privileges."
"Acknowledging change as a 'choice' is a weak position and sends the wrong message."
"There really is no choice, if you think about it. No rational, intelligent person would choose to be an offender."

In addressing these beliefs, there are again varying factors to consider:

1. Assuming that autonomy is selfish or "spoils" the offender is actually a weaker position than acknowledging his or her actual ability to choose. People can always choose to change or not. To comply or not. Insulting them for having a choice only decreases your likelihood of influencing them to make the right decision.

2. It is exhausting to try to convince someone that there isn't a choice, or that your opinion is the only one. This contributes to burnout and frustration on the part of your staff. Stress is debilitating. Too much can easily trigger responses of which staff are not proud. Could the muscle approach become a self-reinforcing loop? Using muscle to convince someone of something he or she doesn't want leads to more discord, which can prompt additional muscle if that's the only tool staff have to use. Staff members' stress levels can increase directiveness and decrease tolerance with offenders in everyday work (Salyers, Hood, Schwartz, Alexander, & Aalsma, 2015). Acknowledging and honoring autonomous decision making may make working with clients not only more effective but also easier.

3. Quite simply—disrespectful treatment is not a sanction. It's just disrespect. Disavowing a person's right of choice is merely disrespectful, and it does little to demonstrate the worth of your view over someone else's. So don't.

4. All change is self-change, or that which comes from within. This isn't surrendering or submission but instead a mind-set that allows

success. The offender is the one responsible for change. Trying to take that away through a power struggle or denial of autonomy makes you responsible for something you cannot control.

5. Courts or other systemic mechanisms will assign consequences for lack of compliance or continued problems. Your approach does little to change that. So why not use an approach that promises more benefit? It would be better to make some progress yet still face problems, than to worsen matters and face exacerbated problems.

PERCEIVED OBSTACLE 3: MI seems too passive.

From an outside view, people may think that MI lacks force or direction. In fact, we have spoken against the use of a directive style. Proponents of this belief may note:

"MI isn't enough; this talk isn't going to do anything."
"MI is so lame! It feels wishy-washy. We need to work on the real issues here."
"How can this relationship-building and affirmation stuff get results?"
"When do you tell them the reality of their situation? That what they're doing hurts people, and that they need to straighten up and get with the program?"

Such concerns are common. The patience and time needed to see results with MI varies widely. While important goals can be accomplished in a matter of minutes (Miller & Rollnick, 2013), with some offenders it may take time. Once again, there are additional factors to consider in responding to these concerns:

1. MI is not necessarily a stand-alone approach, or the only tool in your toolbox. Other methods, approaches, or standardized interventions are available. MI does not preclude the use of these. It is a way of having a conversation that may make other approaches more effective or accessible.

2. Using MI with competency and fidelity involves multiple skills. Practitioners of MI use significant effort; classifying this approach as "passive" is dismissive and inaccurate.

3. The directional aspect of MI is not immediately apparent. Those who give it only superficial consideration may see it as only a "warm" hug-a-thug counseling approach. However, negotiating ambivalence, responding to change talk, and increasing commitment to change are far from passive efforts and require strength from the MI practitioner.

4. While the alternative view might espouse a need for giving advice, doing so often leads nowhere (see Chapter 6). Do you want to be right, or do you want to be effective? Success may depend on your ability to do something other than give advice. Many of your clients have already heard or thought about whatever advice you may have to offer. Many staff understand that giving advice typically does not work. Resolve instead to give offenders something different.

PERCEIVED OBSTACLE 4:
Using MI requires too much time.

Training. Coaching and feedback. Communities of practice. More training. And then you sit and talk with offenders. It may be easy for people to view MI as an additional drain on their time and energy. They may express this in numerous ways:

> "Why listen to all their stories, complaining, and whining? Why not just tell them what to do?"
> "I have a huge caseload. There's no time to do this stuff."
> "I'm so busy that I need to get to the point quickly. But that's not what MI says to do."
> "I know how to do my job. I get good results. I don't need all of this additional training and oversight to tell me what I'm already doing right."

Anyone who works with offenders feels the pressure of limited time and limited resources. It is all too easy to dismiss new efforts if you feel they will compromise time management and effectiveness. However, we hope this volume has made it clear that MI is a practice that can not only improve outcomes but save valuable time in engaging an offender in the conversation. Some other points may be relevant:

1. Time *should* be spent to make our communities safer. Should you miss opportunities to elicit the client's own arguments for change,

you also miss the chance to stop repeat offenses. Too much teaching, advising, and confronting fails to recognize the person's own internal dilemmas and can slow important change conversation.

2. MI may take longer initially in the short run but will pay off in the long run. More investment on the front end leads to less stress and difficulty later.

3. Using MI circumvents the later time spent with confrontation and lecturing, leading to the earlier establishment of genuine communication.

4. Dealing with continued problem behavior also takes time. Investing in proactive efforts to understand and engage with the offender may also save time typically needed for addressing ongoing problems.

5. While you can easily make the situation worse in only a few minutes, you can also improve it in a relatively short period of time. Which would you prefer? If what you want is behavior change and you don't have a lot of time, MI is a good way to go.

PERCEIVED OBSTACLE 5:
If I use MI, my coworkers will look down on me.

This belief contains within it several assumptions related to obstacles we have already discussed. If you think that MI excuses denial, weakens the court's authority, or is passive, it stands to reason that you would fear being viewed in a negative light for using it. However, we hope that by now you're beginning to see how insidious (and incorrect) these beliefs and assumptions are. Still, this one can promote fear and hesitation to use MI even among staff who would otherwise be excited about the approach. What you may hear expressed by such concerned staff includes:

"Everyone will just think I'm naïve or too gullible."
"We're supposed to punish them, not be their friends."
"Offenders will play you, and tough staff don't get taken advantage of."
"Seems like it would damage my reputation. I don't want to always have to explain myself to my colleagues."

As always, there are additional factors to consider:

1. First, it is possible that confrontation may work better with some clients. Still, there's a caveat—while some of us can recall making changes when confronted by someone, think about the person who did it. Was it someone who you respected and who wanted the best for you (e.g., parent, coach, teacher, mentor)? Or was it someone distant and hostile, for whom you lacked respect? Even if a confrontational style or incident of challenge was involved, it was likely impactful because it came from a source you were willing to hear it from.

2. When a staff person indicates willingness to try MI but for fear of stigma or reprisal, it represents the perfect opportunity for you to be supportive of a new direction for your agency. You can take on the role as change agent.

3. There are over 1,000 research studies demonstrating that positive relationships are one of the strongest and most consistent predictors of outcomes across approaches (Orlinsky, Ronnestad & Willutzki, 2004). Holding fast to the idea that offender work is any different is simply being resistant to change oneself.

4. People should have the opportunity to judge for themselves once they are more familiar with the approach and can see it work. Those who think MI lets clients off too easily have likely not tried it.

5. The practice of MI does not negate expectations of compliance and assignment of consequences for violations of rules or court orders. Those who begin to use MI but who fear judgment and condemnation from their colleagues would do well to remember that they still have responsibilities, and that others seeing them enforcing rules will soon begin to drop their criticism of the approach.

> *Those who think MI lets clients off too easily have likely not tried it.*

PERCEIVED OBSTACLE 6:
MI is for everyone; or, relatedly, MI is a cure-all.

We hope that we have convinced you in this text that MI can certainly be of benefit to your agency and the offenders with whom you work. That being said, we don't claim that MI is a magical elixir that will cure the world's ills. With this obstacle, you may hear a variety of beliefs expressed:

> "Whatever happened to 'different strokes for different folks'? This just treats everyone like they're the same."
>
> "This is just another fad—a new idea from people who don't know what it's like to do my job."
>
> "I think it works best to know lots of approaches and methods. Everyone is different, and this will probably only work for those on my caseload who are really easy to talk to already."

Several factors are worth considering in the face of these doubts:

1. MI is an evidence-based practice. Evidence-based approaches have been evaluated in diverse areas, with different clients, by different staff. Further, initial studies on MI with offender populations demonstrate its effectiveness (Anstiss et al., 2011; Council of State Governments Justice Center, 2014), and the use of MI by correctional and criminal justice agency staff has been suggested by the U.S. Department of Justice (Guevara & Solomon, 2009). Is it the end of the search for effective offender approaches? Of course not. It may someday be replaced by something that works even better. But for now, the results are quite promising.

2. The issue of readiness to change is recognized as being important within offender services (Ward, Day, Howells, & Birgden, 2004). MI engages clients in the change process with a focus on increasing readiness to change. Offenders may not always succeed, but at least they are focused on their behaviors and lifestyle choices rather than defending their problem behavior or arguing with staff. This approach places greater emphasis on taking personal responsibility for one's behavior.

The focus of personnel in offender services agencies is currently undergoing a transition (e.g., Serin, Chadwick, & Lloyd, 2015). No longer are those who work with offenders seen as solely agents of supervision, control, or risk management. Instead, their roles are shifting to include actively engaging clients in their work. MI corresponds with these new objectives.

PERCEIVED OBSTACLE 7: This will only work with some offenders, but not the ones I work with.

Interestingly, those who work with specialized populations sometimes develop the mind-set that what works for those "other" offenders will never work for their own. This may be true of personnel whose clients include high-risk offenders, sex offenders, offenders with mental illness, violent offenders, gang members, or others. Certainly, working and specializing with a group of offenders builds expertise. But such expertise should not exclude viable approaches that offer many potential benefits. This attitude may manifest itself in the following kinds of statements:

> "MI is only for low-risk offenders."
> "MI might work for some populations but not *all*. You need to do something different with *this* type of person."
> "I can see how that might work well with other groups, but mine will never go for it."

Once again, consideration of a number of factors may guide your response to such concerns:

1. No matter what population you work with, the mechanisms that propel behavior change remain consistent. This is the reason that MI has such broad applicability to such seemingly different groups (see Chapter 13).

2. Acknowledging personal choice (i.e., autonomy), developing collaborative partnerships, and finding intrinsic reasons for change (i.e., evocation) prove to be even *more* important when working with challenging populations. These are groups that are perhaps harder to reach through other means, or who need a different type of relationship or approach in order to achieve successful outcomes. Their differences and uniqueness may in fact make them *more* likely to benefit from MI. To date, no demographic or diagnostic characteristic has predicted failure to respond to MI.

3. Assessing compliance, instituting sanctions, and monitoring progress will always be a part of offender work, and we do not mean to suggest that you ignore this part of your job. But in thinking about the potential effectiveness of MI with your own clients, what do you have to lose?

CONCLUDING THOUGHTS

MI has surely advanced our understanding of what mobilizes people to examine important changes in their lives. It is an approach that is used with a multitude of different populations, for different presenting problems, and in different settings. For our purposes, it is an approach that can certainly advance our practice with offenders in institutional and community settings. MI is a way of having a conversation with offenders that highlights their humanity and their ambivalence about what may be significant life changes. It guides them through their decision making in a respectful and effective manner. And it allows them to begin their journey in a way that ensures more lasting, meaningful behavior change.

A common theme in this text has been balance. And in fact, it is all about balance. As agents of offender systems, it is perhaps all too easy to become mired in the need to be "right" over the need to remain balanced. But even when you are "right," it may not leave you feeling as if you have succeeded. Being "right" when an offender fails, or when the system administers a harsh punishment, or when your colleagues praise you for your objectivity and stoicism in the face of another unfortunate story—all these may leave you feeling disappointed in your own inability to be an effective agent of change. Instead, perhaps it is time to try something new. MI can bring about balance—between spirit and technique, responsibilities and relationships, and compliance with rules and genuine behavior change. We hope that our discussion has piqued your interest, and has shown you how MI can help you and your agency more effectively accomplish the goals of successful offender rehabilitation and reentry. In adopting the spirit and practice of MI, you are helping not only the offender, but also yourself.

REFERENCES

Alexander, M., Lowenkamp, C. T., & Robinson, C. R. (2013). A tale of two innovations: Motivational interviewing and core correctional practices in United States probation. In P. Ugwudike & P. Raynor (Eds.), *What works in offender compliance: International perspectives and evidence-based practices* (pp. 242–255). London: Palgrave Macmillan.

Alexander, M., VanBenschoten, S. W., & Walters, S. T. (2008). Motivational interviewing training in criminal justice: Development of a model plan. *Federal Probation, 72,* 61–66.

Amrhein, P. C., Miller, W. R., Yahne, C. E., Palmer, M., & Fulcher, L. (2003). Client commitment language during motivational interviewing predicts drug use outcomes. *Journal of Consulting and Clinical Psychology, 71*(5), 862–878.

Anderson, H., & Goolishian, H. (1992). The client is the expert: A not knowing approach to therapy. In S. McNamee & K. J. Gergen (Eds.), *Social construction and the therapeutic process* (pp. 117–136). London: Sage.

Andrews, D. A., Bonta, J., & Hoge, R. D. (1990). Classification for effective rehabilitation: Rediscovering psychology. *Criminal Justice and Behavior, 17*(1), 19–52.

Andrews, D. A., & Carvell, C. (1998). *Core correctional training–core correctional supervision and counseling: Theory, research, assessment and practice.* Unpublished training manual, Carleton University, Ottawa, Canada.

Andrews, D. A., & Kiessling, J. J. (1980). Program structure and effective correctional practice: A summary of CaVic research. In R. Ross & P. Gendreau (Eds.), *Effective correctional treatment* (pp. 439–463). Toronto, Ontario, Canada: Butterworths.

Anstiss, B., Polaschek, D. L., & Wilson, M. (2011). A brief motivational interviewing intervention with prisoners: When you lead a horse to water, can it drink for itself? *Psychology, Crime and Law, 17*(8), 689–710.

Apodaca, T. R., & Longabaugh, R. (2009). Mechanisms of change in motivational interviewing: A review and preliminary evaluation of the evidence. *Addiction, 104*(5), 705–715.

Arkowitz, H., Miller, W. R., & Rollnick, S. (Eds.). (2015). *Motivational interviewing in the treatment of psychological problems.* New York: Guilford Press.

Armstrong, K. (2010). *Twelve steps to a compassionate life.* New York: Knopf.

Bachelor, A., & Horvath, A. (1999). The therapeutic relationship. In M. Hubble, B. L. Duncan, & S. D. Miller (Eds.), *The heart and soul of change: What works in therapy* (pp. 143–178). Washington, DC: American Psychological Association.

Baer, J. S., Rosengren, D. B., Dunn, C. W., Wells, E. A., Ogle, R. L., & Hartzler, B. (2004). An evaluation of workshop training in motivational interviewing for addiction and mental health clinicians. *Drug and Alcohol Dependence, 73*(1), 99–106.

Balslev, A., & Evers, D. (2009). *Compassion in the world's religions: Envisioning human solidarity.* Berlin: LIT Verlag.

Bamatter, W., Carroll, K. M., Añez, L. M., Paris, M., Ball, S. A., Nich, C., et al. (2010). Informal discussions in substance abuse treatment sessions with Spanish-speaking clients. *Journal of Substance Abuse Treatment, 39*(4), 353–363.

Bar, M., Neta, M., & Linz, H. (2006). Very first impressions. *Emotion, 6*(2), 269–278.

Barry, M. (2007). Listening and learning: The reciprocal relationship between worker and client. *Probation Journal, 54*(4), 407–422.

Berg, I. K. (1994). *Family based services: A solution focused approach.* New York: Norton.

Berg, I. K., & Kelly, S. (2000). *Building solutions in child protective services.* New York: Norton.

Bernard, R. M., Abrami, P. C., Lou, Y., Borokhovski, E., Wade, A., Wozney, L., et al. (2004). How does distance education compare with classroom instruction?: A meta-analysis of the empirical literature. *Review of Educational Research, 74,* 379–439.

Birgden, A. (2004). Therapeutic jurisprudence and responsivity: Finding the will and the way in offender rehabilitation. *Psychology, Crime and Law, 10*(3), 283–295.

Bogue, B., Campbell, N., Carey, M., Clawson, E., Faust, D., Florio, K., et al. (2004). *Implementing evidence-based practice in community corrections: The principles of effective intervention.* Washington, DC: National Institute of Corrections.

Bogue, B., Diebel, J., & O'Connor, T. (2008). Combining officer supervision skills: A new model for increasing success in community corrections. *Perspectives: Journal of the American Probation and Parole Association, 32,* 31–45.

Bogue, B., Pampel, F., & Pasini-Hill, D. (2013). Progress toward motivational interviewing proficiency in corrections: Results of a Colorado staff development program. *Justice Research and Policy, 15*(1), 37–66.

Bohart, A. C., & Tallman, K. (1999). *How clients make therapy work: The process of active self-healing.* Washington, DC: American Psychological Association.

Bonk, C. J., & Graham, C. R. (2006). *The handbook of blended learning.* San Francisco: Pfeiffer.

Bonta, J., & Andrews, D. A. (2003). A commentary on Ward and Stewart's model of human needs. *Psychology Crime and Law, 9*(3), 215–218.

Bonta, J., & Andrews, D. A. (2007). Risk–need–responsivity model for offender assessment and rehabilitation. *Rehabilitation, 6,* 1–22.

Bonta, J., Bourgon, G., Rugge, T., Scott, T. L., Yessine, A. K., Gutierrez, L. K., et al. (2010). *The strategic training initiative in community supervision: Risk–need–responsivity in the real world.* Ottawa, Ontario: Public Safety Canada.

Bonta, J., Rugge, T., Scott, T. L., Bourgon, G., & Yessine, A. K. (2008). Exploring the black box of community supervision. *Journal of Offender Rehabilitation, 47*(3), 248–270.

Bordin, E. S. (1979). The generalizability of the psychoanalytic concept of the working alliance. *Psychotherapy: Theory, Research and Practice, 16*(3), 252.

Botelho, R. J. (2004) *Motivational practice: Promoting healthy habits and self-care of chronic diseases.* Rochester, NY: MHH Publications.

Bozarth, J. (2010). *Social media for trainers: Techniques for enhancing and extending learning.* San Francisco: Wiley.

Brown, J. M., & Miller, W. R. (1993). Impact of motivational interviewing on participation and outcome in residential alcoholism treatment. *Psychology of Addictive Behaviors, 7*(4), 211–218.

Burke, B. L., Arkowitz, H., & Dunn, C. (2002). The efficacy of motivational interviewing and its adaptations: What we know so far. In W. R. Miller & S. Rollnick, *Motivational interviewing: Preparing people for change* (2nd ed., pp. 217–250). New York: Guilford Press.

Burnett, R., & McNeill, F. (2005). The place of the officer–offender relationship in assisting offenders to desist from crime. *Probation Journal, 52*(3), 221–242.

Bush, J., Glick, B., Taymans, J., & Guevara, M. L. (2011). *Thinking for a change: Integrated cognitive behavior change program.* Washington, DC: National Institute of Corrections.

Butler, C. C., Rollnick, S., Cohen, D., Bachmann, M., Russell, I., & Stott, N. (1999). Motivational consulting versus brief advice for smokers in general practice: A randomized trial. *British Journal of General Practice, 49*(445), 611–616.

Camp, J. R. (2002). *Start with no: The negotiating tools that the pros don't want you to know.* New York: Crown.

Carlbring, P., Jonsson, J., Josephson, H., & Forsberg, L. (2010). Motivational interviewing versus cognitive behavioral group therapy in the treatment of problem and pathological gambling: A randomized controlled trial. *Cognitive Behaviour Therapy, 39*(2), 92–103.

Carlisle, L. (2014). *Motivational interviewing in dentistry: Helping people become healthier.* Carbondale, CO: Adjuvant New Media.

Christensen, A., & Jacobson, N. S. (1994). Who (or what) can do psychotherapy: The status and challenge of nonprofessional therapies. *Psychological Science, 5*(1), 8–14.

Clark, M. D. (2005). Motivational interviewing for probation staff: Increasing the readiness to change. *Federal Probation, 69*(2), 22–28.

Clark, M. D. (2006). Entering the business of behavior change: Motivational interviewing for probation staff. *Perspectives, 30*(1), 38–45.

Clark, M. D. (2008). Moving from compliance to behavior change: Motivational interviewing and the juvenile court. *Juvenile and Family Justice Today, 17*(3), 22–23.

Clark, M. D. (2009). The strengths perspective in criminal justice. *The strengths perspective in social work practice.* New York: Longman.

Clark, M. D., Walters, S., Gingerich, R., & Meltzer, M. (2006). Motivational interviewing for probation officers: Tipping the balance toward change. *Federal Probation, 70*(1), 38–44.

Clark, R. C., & Mayer, R. E. (2007). *e-learning and the science of instruction.* San Francisco: Pfeiffer.

Clark, R. E. (1994). Media will never influence learning. *Educational Technology Research and Development, 42*(2), 21–30.

Clark, R. E. (1999). Yin and yang cognitive motivational processes operating in multimedia learning environments. In J. van Merrienböer (Ed.), *Cognition and multimedia design* (pp. 73–107). Herleen, The Netherlands: Open University Press.

Clark, R. E., Bewley, W. L., & O'Neil, H. (2006). Heuristics for selecting distance or classroom settings for courses. In H. O'Neil & R. Perez (Eds.), *Web-based learning: Theory, research and practice* (pp. 133–142). Mahwah, NJ: Erlbaum.

Clarke, R. V. (1995). Situational crime prevention (pp. 91–150). In M. Tonry & D. P. Farrington (Eds.), *Building a safer society: Strategic approaches to crime prevention.* Chicago: University of Chicago Press.

Clear, T. R., & Frost, N. (2013). *The punishment imperative.* New York: New York University Press.

Clifford, D., & Curtis, L. (2016). *Motivational interviewing in nutrition and fitness.* New York: Guilford Press.

Council of State Governments Justice Center. (2014). *Reducing recidivism: States deliver results.* New York: Author.

Cullen, F. T. (2007). Make rehabilitation corrections' guiding paradigm. *Criminology and Public Policy, 6*(4), 717–727.

Dalai Lama, & Vreeland, N. (2001). *An open heart: Practicing compassion in everyday life.* Boston: Little, Brown.

Deci, E. L., & Ryan, R. M. (1985). *Intrinsic motivation and self-determination in human behavior.* New York: Plenum Press.

Dia, D. A., Simmons, C. A., Oliver, M. A., & Cooper, R. L. (2009). Motivational interviewing for perpetrators of intimate partner violence. In P. Lehmann & C. A. Simmons (Eds.), *Strengths-based batterer intervention: A new paradigm in ending family violence* (pp. 87–111). New York: Springer.

Dickinson, D. M., Edmundson, E., & Tomlin, K. (2006). Implementing motivational interviewing: Lessons from clinical experiences. *Journal of Teaching in the Addictions, 5*(2), 39–57.

DiClemente, C. C. (2003). *Addiction and change: How addictions develop and addicted people recover.* New York: Guilford Press.

Diskin, K. M., & Hodgins, D. C. (2009). A randomized controlled trial of a single session motivational intervention for concerned gamblers. *Behaviour Research and Therapy, 47*(5), 382–388.

Dowden, C., & Andrews, D. A. (1999). What works for female offenders: A meta-analytic review. *Crime and Delinquency, 45*(4), 438–452.

Dowden, C., & Andrews, D. A. (2000). Effective correctional treatment and violent reoffending: A meta-analysis. *Canadian Journal of Criminology, 42,* 449–467.

Dowden, C., & Andrews, D. A. (2004). The importance of staff practice in delivering effective correctional treatment: A meta-analytic review of core correctional practice. *International Journal of Offender Therapy and Comparative Criminology, 48*(2), 203–214.

Duncan, B. L., Miller, S. D., Sparks, J. A., Claud, D. A., Reynolds, L. R., Brown, J., et al. (2003). The Session Rating Scale: Preliminary psychometric properties of a "working" alliance measure. *Journal of Brief Therapy, 3*(1), 3–12.

Duncan, B., Miller, S., Wampold, B., & Hubble, M. (2009). *The heart and soul of change: Delivering what works in therapy* (2nd ed.). Washington, DC: American Psychological Association.

Duncan, E., Best, C., & Hagen, S. (2010, January 20). Shared decision making interventions for people with mental health conditions. *Cochrane Database of Systematic Reviews, 1,* CD007297.

Engle, D. E., & Arkowitz, H. (2006). *Ambivalence in psychotherapy: Facilitating readiness to change.* New York: Guilford Press.

Farbring, C. Å., & Johnson, W. R. (2008). Motivational interviewing in the correctional system: An attempt to implement motivational interviewing in criminal justice. In H. Arkowitz, H. A. Westra, W. R. Miller, & S. Rollnick (Eds.), *Motivational interviewing in the treatment of psychological problems* (pp. 304–323). New York: Guilford Press.

Farrall, S. (2002). *Rethinking what works with offenders: Probation, social context, and desistance from crime.* Portland, OR: Willan.

Feldstein, S. W., & Ginsburg, J. I. D. (2007). Sex, drugs, and rock 'n' rolling with resistance: Motivational interviewing in juvenile justice settings. In D. W. Springer & A. R. Roberts (Eds.), *Handbook of forensic mental health with victims and offenders: Assessment, treatment, and research* (pp. 247–271). New York: Springer.

Festervan, E. (2000). *Survival guide for new probation officers.* Lanham, MD: American Correctional Association.

Fixsen, D. L., & Blase, K. A. (2007, November). *National Implementation Research Network.* Paper presented at the NCTI Technology Innovators Conference, Washington, DC.

Fixsen, D. L., Blase, K. A., Horner, R. H., & Sugai, G. (2009). *Developing the capacity for scaling up the effective use of evidence-based programs in state departments of education.* Concept paper, University of North Carolina at Chapel Hill, University of Oregon, and University of Connecticut.

Fixsen, D. L., Naoom, S. F., Blase, K. A., Friedman, R. M., & Wallace, F. (2005). *Implementation research: A synthesis of the literature* (FMHI #231). Tampa: University of South Florida, Louis de la Parte Florida Mental Health Institute, National Implementation Research Network.

Forsberg, L., Ernst, D., & Farbring, C. Å. (2011). Learning motivational interviewing in a real-life setting: A randomised controlled trial in the Swedish Prison Service. *Criminal Behaviour and Mental Health, 21*(3), 177–188.

Frey, J. (2008). *Motivational interviewing and behavioral compliance in chronic pain patients: A treatment outcome study.* Unpublished doctoral dissertation, George Fox University, Newberg, OR.

Gandhi, M. (1978). *Hindu dharma.* New Delhi, India: Orient Paperbacks.

Gasser, U., & Palfrey, J. (2008). *Born digital: Connecting with a global generation of digital natives.* New York: Perseus.

Ginsburg, J. I. D., Mann, R. E., Rotgers, F., & Weekes, J. R. (2002). Motivational interviewing with criminal justice populations. In W. R. Miller & S. Rollnick, *Motivational interviewing: Preparing people for change* (2nd ed., pp. 333–346). New York: Guilford Press.

Gladwell, M. (2013). *David and Goliath: Underdogs, misfits, and the art of battling giants.* Boston: Little, Brown.

Gleicher, L., Manchak, S. M., & Cullen, F. T. (2013). Creating a supervision tool kit: How to improve probation and parole. *Federal Probation, 77*(1), 22–27.

Glynn, L. H., & Moyers, T. B. (2012). Manual for the Client Language Easy Rating (CLEAR) Coding System. Retrieved from *http://casaa.unm.edu/download/CLEAR.pdf.*

Gordon, T. G. (1970). *Parent effectiveness training: The "no-lose" program for raising responsible children.* New York: Wyden.

Grodin, J. P. (2006). *Assessing therapeutic change mechanisms in motivational interviewing using the articulated thoughts in simulated situations paradigm.* Doctoral dissertation, University of Southern California, Los Angeles, CA.

Grossman, P., Niemann, L., Schmidt, S., & Walach, H. (2004). Mindfulness-based stress reduction and health benefits: A meta-analysis. *Journal of Psychosomatic Research, 57*(1), 35–43.

Guevara, M., & Solomon, E. (2009). *Implementing evidence-based policy and practice in community corrections* (2nd ed.). Washington, DC: National Institute of Corrections.

Harkins, L., & Beech, A. R. (2007). A review of the factors that can influence the effectiveness of sexual offender treatment: Risk, need, responsivity, and process issues. *Aggression and Violent Behavior, 12*(6), 615–627.

Harper, R., & Hardy, S. (2000). An evaluation of motivational interviewing as a method of intervention with clients in a probation setting. *British Journal of Social Work, 30*(3), 393–400.

Harris, M. K. (2005). In search of common ground: The importance of theoretical orientations in criminology and criminal justice. *Criminology and Public Policy, 4,* 311–328.

Hartzler, B., & Espinosa, E. M. (2011). Moving criminal justice organizations toward adoption of evidence-based practice via advanced workshop training in motivational interviewing: A research note. *Criminal Justice Policy Review, 22*(2), 235–253.

Hawkins, D. M. (1998). An invitation to join in difficulty: Realizing the deeper promise of group psychotherapy. *International Journal of Group Psychotherapy, 48*(4), 423–438.

Hohman, M. (Ed.). (2012). *Motivational interviewing in social work practice.* New York: Guilford Press.

Hohman, M., Doran, N., & Koutsenok, I. (2009). Motivational interviewing training for juvenile correctional staff in California: One year initial outcomes. *Journal of Offender Rehabilitation, 48*(7), 635–648.

Hohman, M., & Matulich, W. (2010). Initial validation of the motivational interviewing measure of staff interaction. *Alcoholism Treatment Quarterly, 28*(2), 230–238.

Hubble, M. A., Duncan, B. L., & Miller, S. D. (1999). *The heart and soul of change: What works in therapy.* Washington, DC: American Psychological Association.

Jacobson, N. S., & Gurman, J. S. (Eds.). (1995). *Clinical handbook of couple therapy* (2nd ed.). New York: Guilford Press.

Janis, I. L. (1972). *Victims of groupthink: A psychological study of foreign-policy decisions and fiascoes.* Oxford, UK: Houghton Mifflin.

Jensen, C. D., Cushing, C. C., Aylward, B. S., Craig, J. T., Sorell, D. M., & Steele, R. G. (2011). Effectiveness of motivational interviewing interventions for adolescent substance use behavior change: A meta-analytic review. *Journal of Consulting and Clinical Psychology, 79*(4), 433–440.

Joplin, L., Bogue, B., Campbell, N., Carey, M., Clawson, E., Faust, D., et al. (2004). *Using an integrated model to implement evidence-based practices in corrections.* Boston: Crime and Justice Institute.

Kaczynski, D. (2007). *Public mental health services: One family's perspective.* Keynote presentation at the conference of the National Association of State Mental Health Program Directors, Forensic Division, San Antonio, TX.

Karno, M. P., & Longabaugh, R. (2004). What do we know?: Process analysis and the search for a better understanding of Project MATCH's anger-by-treatment matching effect. *Journal of Studies on Alcohol, 65*(4), 501–512.

Karno, M. P., & Longabaugh, R. (2005a). An examination of how therapist directiveness interacts with patient anger and reactance to predict alcohol use. *Journal of Studies on Alcohol, 66*(6), 825–832.

Karno, M. P., & Longabaugh, R. (2005b). Less directiveness by therapists improves drinking outcomes of reactant clients in alcoholism treatment. *Journal of Consulting and Clinical Psychology, 73*(2), 262–267.

Karno, M. P., Longabaugh, R., & Herbeck, D. (2009). Patient reactance as a moderator of the effect of therapist structure on posttreatment alcohol use. *Journal of Studies on Alcohol and Drugs, 70*(6), 929–936.

Kistenmacher, B. R., & Weiss, R. L. (2008). Motivational interviewing as a mechanism for change in men who batter: A randomized controlled trial. *Violence and Victims, 23*(5), 558–570.

Knight, K. M., McGowan, L., Dickens, C., & Bundy, C. (2006). A systematic review of motivational interviewing in physical health care settings. *British Journal of Health Psychology, 11*(2), 319–332.

Lewis, S. (2014). Learning from success and failure: Deconstructing the working relationship within probation practice and exploring its impact on probationers, using a collaborative approach. *Probation Journal, 61*(2), 161–175.

Longabaugh, R., Zweben, A., Locastro, J. S., & Miller, W. R. (2005). Origins, issues and options in the development of the combined behavioral intervention. *Journal of Studies on Alcohol and Drugs, 66*(Suppl. 15), 179–187.

Lowenkamp, C. T., Holsinger, A. M., Robinson, C. R., & Cullen, F. T. (2012). When a person isn't a data point: Making evidence-based practice work. *Federal Probation, 76,* 11–21.

Lundahl, B., & Burke, B. L. (2009). The effectiveness and applicability of motivational interviewing: A practice-friendly review of four meta-analyses. *Journal of Clinical Psychology, 65*(11), 1232–1245.

Mace, C. (2007). *Mindfulness and mental health: Therapy, theory and science.* East Sussex, UK: Routledge.

Martino, S., Ball, S., Nich, C., Frankforter, T. L., & Carroll, K. M. (2009). Correspondence of motivational enhancement treatment integrity ratings among therapists, supervisors, and observers. *Psychotherapy Research, 19*(2), 181–193.

Maruna, S., & Immarigeon, R. (2004). *After crime and punishment: Pathways to ex-offender reintegration.* Portland, OR: Willan.

Mayer, R. E. (Ed.). (2005). *The Cambridge handbook of multimedia learning.* New York: Cambridge University Press.

McGrath, R. J., Cumming, G., & Holt, J. (2002). Collaboration among sex offender treatment providers and probation and parole officers: The beliefs and behaviors of treatment providers. *Sexual Abuse: A Journal of Research and Treatment, 14,* 49–65.

McMurran, M. (2002). *Motivating offenders to change: A guide to enhancing engagement in therapy.* West Sussex, UK: Wiley.

McMurran, M. (2009). Motivational interviewing with offenders: A systematic review. *Legal and Criminological Psychology, 14*(1), 83–100.

McNeill, F. (2012). Four forms of "offender" rehabilitation: Towards an interdisciplinary perspective. *Legal and Criminological Psychology, 17*(1), 18–36.

Mendel, E., & Hipkins, J. (2002). Motivating learning disabled offenders with alcohol-related problems: A pilot study. *British Journal of Learning Disabilities, 30*(4), 153–158.

Meyers, R. J., & Wolfe, B. L. (2004). *Get your loved one sober: Alternatives to nagging, pleading and threatening.* Center City, MN: Hazelden.

Miller, W. R. (1983). Motivational interviewing with problem drinkers. *Behavioural Psychotherapy, 11*(2), 147–172.

Miller, W. R. (Ed.). (1999). *Enhancing motivation for change in substance abuse treatment* (Treatment Improvement Protocol [TIP] Series, No. 35). Rockville, MD: Center for Substance Abuse.

Miller, W. R. (2000). Rediscovering fire: Small interventions, large effects. *Psychology of Addictive Behaviors, 14,* 6–18.

Miller, W. R. (Ed.). (2004). *COMBINE Monograph Series: Vol. 1. Combined behavioral intervention manual: A clinical research guide for therapists treating people with alcohol abuse and dependence.* Bethesda, MD: National Institute on Alcohol Abuse and Alcoholism.

Miller, W. R., Benefield, R. G., & Tonigan, J. S. (1993). Enhancing motivation for change in problem drinking: A controlled comparison of two therapist styles. *Journal of Consulting and Clinical Psychology, 61*(3), 455–461.

Miller, W. R., Meyers, R. J., & Tonigan, J. S. (1999). Engaging the unmotivated in treatment for alcohol problems: A comparison of three strategies for intervention through family members. *Journal of Consulting and Clinical Psychology, 67*(5), 688–697.

Miller, W. R., & Mount, K. A. (2001). A small study of training in motivational interviewing: Does one workshop change clinician and client behavior? *Behavioural and Cognitive Psychotherapy, 29*(4), 457–471.

Miller, W. R., & Moyers, T. B. (2006). Eight stages in learning motivational interviewing. *Journal of Teaching in the Addictions, 5,* 3–17.

Miller, W. R., & Rollnick, S. (1991). *Motivational interviewing: Preparing people to change addictive behavior.* New York: Guilford Press.

Miller, W. R., & Rollnick, S. (2002). *Motivational interviewing: Preparing people for change* (2nd ed.). New York: Guilford Press.

Miller, W. R., & Rollnick, S. (2003). Motivational interviewing: Preparing people for change. *Journal for Healthcare Quality, 25*(3), 46.

Miller, W. R., & Rollnick, S. (2004). Talking oneself into change: Motivational interviewing, stages of change, and therapeutic process. *Journal of Cognitive Psychotherapy, 18*(4), 299–308.

Miller, W. R., & Rollnick, S. (2009). Ten things that motivational interviewing is not. *Behavioural and Cognitive Psychotherapy, 37*(2), 129–140.

Miller, W. R., & Rollnick, S. (2013). *Motivational interviewing: Helping people change* (3rd ed.). New York: Guilford Press.

Miller, W. R., Yahne, C. E., Moyers, T. B., Martinez, J., & Pirritano, M. (2004). A randomized trial of methods to help clinicians learn motivational interviewing. *Journal of Consulting and Clinical Psychology, 72*(6), 1050–1062.

Moyers, T. B., & Martin, T. (2006). Therapist influence on client language during motivational interviewing sessions. *Journal of Substance Abuse Treatment, 30*(3), 245–251.

Moyers, T. B., Martin, T., Catley, D., Harris, K. J., & Ahluwalia, J. S. (2003). Assessing the integrity of motivational interventions: Reliability of the Motivational Interviewing Skills Code. *Behavioural and Cognitive Psychotherapy, 31,* 177–184.

Moyers, T. B., Rowell, L. N., Manuel, J. K., Ernst, D., & Houck, J. M. (2016). The Motivational Interviewing Treatment Integrity code (MITI 4): Rationale, preliminary reliability and validity. *Journal of Substance Abuse Treatment, 65,* 36–42.

Murphy, C. M., & Maiuro, R. D. (2009). *Motivational interviewing and stages of change in intimate partner violence.* New York: Springer.

Musser, P. H., & Murphy, C. M. (2009). Motivational interviewing with perpetrators of intimate partner abuse. *Journal of Clinical Psychology, 65*(11), 1218–1231.

Musser, P. H., Semiatin, J. N., Taft, C. T., & Murphy, C. M. (2008). Motivational interviewing as a pregroup intervention for partner-violent men. *Violence and Victims, 23*(5), 539–557.

Nhat Hanh, T. (1999). *The heart of the Buddha's teaching: Transforming suffering into peace, joy, and liberation.* New York: Random House.

Norcross, J. C. (Ed.). (2002). *Psychotherapy relationships that work: Therapist contributions and responsiveness to patients.* New York: Oxford University Press.

Orlinsky, D. E., Ronnestad, M. H., & Willutzki, U. (2004). Fifty years of psychotherapy process-outcome research: Continuity and change. In M. Lambert (Ed.), *Bergin and Garfield's handbook of psychotherapy and behavior change* (5th ed., pp. 307–389). New York: Wiley.

Patterson, G. R., & Chamberlain, P. (1994). A functional analysis of resistance during parent training therapy. *Clinical Psychology: Science and Practice, 1*(1), 53–70.

Peele, S., Brodsky, A., & Arnold, M. (1991). *The truth about addiction and recovery: The life process program for outgrowing destructive habits.* New York: Simon & Schuster.

Petry, N. M., Weinstock, J., Ledgerwood, D. M., & Morasco, B. (2008). A randomized trial of brief interventions for problem and pathological gamblers. *Journal of Consulting and Clinical Psychology, 76*(2), 318–328.

Polaschek, D. L. (2012). An appraisal of the risk–need–responsivity (RNR) model of offender rehabilitation and its application in correctional treatment. *Legal and Criminological Psychology, 17*(1), 1–17.

Prochaska, J. O., & DiClemente, C. C. (1982). Transtheoretical therapy: Toward a more integrative model of change. *Psychotherapy: Theory, Research, and Practice, 19*(3), 276–288.

Prochaska, J. O., & DiClemente, C. C. (1992). Stages of change in the modification of problem behaviors. In M. Hersen, R. M. Eisler, & P. M. Miller (Eds.), *Progress in behavior modification* (pp. 184–214). Sycamore, IL: Sycamore Press.

Prochaska, J. O., DiClemente, C. C., & Norcross, J. C. (1992a). In search of how people change: Applications to addictive behaviors. *American Psychologist, 47*(9), 1102–1114.

Prochaska, J. O., DiClemente, C. C., & Norcross, J. C. (1992b). In search of the structure of change. In *Self change* (pp. 87–114). New York: Springer.

Rasmussen, L. A., Hughes, M. J., & Murray, C. A. (2008). Applying motivational interviewing in a domestic violence shelter: A pilot study evaluating the training of shelter staff. *Journal of Aggression, Maltreatment and Trauma, 17*(3), 296–317.

Rau, J., Ehlebracht-König, I., & Petermann, F. (2008). Impact of a motivational intervention on coping with chronic pain: Results of a controlled efficacy study. *Schmerz, 22*(5), 575–578.

Robinson, C. R., VanBenschoten, S., Alexander, M., & Lowenkamp, C. T. (2011). A random (almost) study of staff training aimed at reducing re-arrest (STARR): Reducing recidivism through intentional design. *Federal Probation, 75,* 57–63.

Rogers, C. R. (1951). *Client-centered therapy: Its current practice, implications and theory.* Boston: Houghton Mifflin.

Rogers, C. R. (1957). The necessary and sufficient conditions of therapeutic personality change. *Journal of Consulting Psychology, 21,* 95–103.

Rogers, C. R. (1965). The therapeutic relationship: Recent theory and research. *Australian Journal of Psychology, 17*(2), 95–108.

Rogers, C. R. (1986). Carl Rogers on the development of the person-centered approach. *Person-Centered Review, 1*(3), 257–259.

Rollnick, S., Kaplan, S. G., & Rutschman, R. (2016). *Motivational interviewing in schools: Conversations to improve behavior and learning.* New York: Guilford Press.

Rollnick, S., & Miller, W. R. (1995). What is motivational interviewing? *Behavioural and Cognitive Psychotherapy, 23*(4), 325–334.

Rosengren, D. B., Hartzler, B., Baer, J. S., Wells, E. A., & Dunn, C. W. (2008). The Video Assessment of Simulated Encounters—Revised (VASE-R): Reliability and validity of a revised measure of motivational interviewing skills. *Drug and Alcohol Dependence, 97*(1), 130–138.

Rubino, G., Barker, C., Roth, T., & Fearon, P. (2000). Therapist empathy and depth of interpretation in response to potential alliance ruptures: The role of therapist and patient attachment styles. *Psychotherapy Research, 10*(4), 408–420.

Saarni, C., & Lewis, M. (1993). Deceit and illusion in human affairs. In M. Lewis & C. Saarni (Eds.), *Lying and deception in everyday life* (pp. 1–29). New York: Guilford Press.

Safran, J. D., Crocker, P., McMain, S., & Murray, P. (1990). Therapeutic alliance rupture as a therapy event for empirical investigation. *Psychotherapy: Theory, Research, Practice, Training, 27*(2), 154–165.

Salyers, M. P., Hood, B. J., Schwartz, K., Alexander, A. O., & Aalsma, M. C. (2015). The experience, impact, and management of professional burnout among probation officers in juvenile justice settings. *Journal of Offender Rehabilitation, 54*(3), 175–193.

Salzberg, S. (1995). *Lovingkindness: The revolutionary art of happiness.* Boston: Shambhala.

Samenow, S. E. (1978). The criminal personality: New concepts and new procedures for change. *Humanist, 38,* 16–19.

Sellman, J. D., Sullivan, P. F., Dore, G. M., Adamson, S. J., & MacEwan, I. (2001). A randomized controlled trial of motivational enhancement therapy (MET) for mild to moderate alcohol dependence. *Journal of Studies on Alcohol, 62*(3), 389–396.

Serin, R. C., Chadwick, N., & Lloyd, C. D. (2015). Dynamic risk and protective factors. *Psychology, Crime and Law, 22,* 1–44.

Shapiro, S. L., & Carlson, L. E. (2009). *The art and science of mindfulness: Integrating mindfulness into psychology and the helping professions.* Washington, DC: American Psychological Association.

Sigmon, S. T., & Snyder, C. R. (1993). Looking at oneself in a rose-colored mirror: The role of excuses in the negotiation of a personal reality. In M. Lewis & C. Saarni (Eds.), *Lying and deception in everyday life* (pp. 148–165). New York: Guilford Press.

Sinha, R., Easton, C., Renee-Aubin, L., & Carroll, K. M. (2003). Engaging young probation-referred marijuana-abusing individuals in treatment: A pilot trial. *American Journal on Addictions, 12*(4), 314–323.

Slavet, J. D., Stein, L. A., Klein, J. L., Colby, S. M., Barnett, N. P., & Monti, P. M. (2005). Piloting the family check-up with incarcerated adolescents and their parents. *Psychological Services, 2*(2), 123–132.

Snyder, C. R. (1994). *The psychology of hope.* New York: Free Press.

Soria, R., Legido, A., Escolano, C., Lopez Yeste, A., & Montoya, J. (2006). A randomised controlled trial of motivational interviewing for smoking cessation. *British Journal of General Practice, 56*(531), 768–774.

Spiller, V., & Guelfi, G. P. (2007). Motivational interviewing in the criminal justice system. In G. Tober & D. Raistrick (Eds.), *Motivational dialogue: Preparing addiction professionals for motivational interviewing practice* (pp. 151–162). New York: Routledge.

Steinberg, M. P., & Miller, W. R. (2015). *Motivational interviewing in diabetes care.* New York: Guilford Press.

Strupp, H. H., & Hadley, S. W. (1979). Specific vs nonspecific factors in psychotherapy: A controlled study of outcome. *Archives of General Psychiatry, 36*(10), 1125–1136.

Substance Abuse and Mental Health Services Administration. (2008). National registry of evidence-based programs and practices. Retrieved from *www.nrepp.samhsa.gov.*

Taxman, F. S., Cropsey, K. L., Melnick, G., & Perdoni, M. L. (2008). COD services in community correctional settings: An examination of organizational factors that affect service delivery. *Behavioral Sciences and the Law, 26*(4), 435–455.

Thevos, A. K., Quick, R. E., & Yanjuli, V. (2000). Motivational interviewing enhances the adoption of water disinfection practices in Zambia. *Health Promotion International, 15,* 207–214.

Tolle, E. (1999). *The power of now: A guide to spiritual enlightenment.* Novato, CA: Namaste.

Tomlin, K. M., & Richardson, H. (2004). *Motivational interviewing and stages of change: Integrating best practices for substance abuse professionals.* Center City, MN: Hazelden Publishing & Educational Services.

Trotter, C. (1996). The impact of different supervision practices in community corrections: Cause for optimism. *Australian and New Zealand Journal of Criminology, 29*(1), 1–19.

Turmel, W. (2011). *10 steps to successful virtual presentations.* Alexandria, VA: American Society for Training and Development.

Turnell, A., & Edwards, S. (1999). *Signs of safety: A solution oriented approach to child protection casework.* New York: Norton.

University of Cincinnati Corrections Institute. (n.d.). The EPICS model. Retrieved from *www.uc.edu.*

Vasilaki, E. I., Hosier, S. G., & Cox, W. M. (2006). The efficacy of motivational interviewing as a brief intervention for excessive drinking: A meta-analytic review. *Alcohol and Alcoholism, 41*(3), 328–335.

Viets, V. L., Walker, D. D., & Miller, W. R. (2002). What is motivation to change?: A scientific analysis. In M. McMurran (Ed.), *Motivating offenders to change: A guide to enhancing engagement in therapy* (pp. 15–30). West Sussex, UK: Wiley.

Waldron, H. B., Miller, W. R., & Tonigan, J. S. (2001). Client anger as a predictor of differential response to treatment. In R. Longabaugh & P. W. Wirtz (Eds.), *Project MATCH hypotheses: Results and causal chain analyses* (Vol. 8, pp. 134–148). Bethesda, MD: National Institute on Alcohol Abuse and Alcoholism.

Walters, S. T., Clark, M. D., Gingerich, R., & Meltzer, M. L. (2007). *Motivating offenders to change: A guide for probation and parole.* Washington DC: National Institute of Corrections, U.S. Department of Justice.

Walters, S. T., Ogle, R. L., & Martin, J. E. (2002). Perils and possibilities of group-based MI. In W. R. Miller & S. Rollnick, *Motivational interviewing: Preparing people to change* (2nd ed., pp. 377–390). New York: Guilford Press.

Walters, S. T., Vader, A. M., Nguyen, N., Harris, T. R., & Eells, J. (2010). Motivational interviewing as a supervision strategy in probation: A randomized effectiveness trial. *Journal of Offender Rehabilitation, 49*(5), 309–323.

Ward, T., Day, A., Howells, K., & Birgden, A. (2004). The multifactor offender readiness model. *Aggression and Violent Behavior, 9*(6), 645–673.

Ward, T., & Maruna, S. (2007). *Rehabilitation: Beyond the risk paradigm.* New York: Routledge.

White, W. L., & Miller, W. R. (2007). The use of confrontation in addiction treatment: History, science, and time for change. *Counselor, 8*(4), 12–30.

Yochelson, S., & Samenow, S. E. (1977). A new horizon for total change of the criminal. In *The criminal personality: Vol. 2. The change process* (pp. 3–18). New York: Jason Aronson.

Yu, M., Saleem, M., & Gonzalez, C. (2014). Developing trust: First impressions and experience. *Journal of Economic Psychology, 43*, 16–29.

INDEX

Note. "f " or "t" following a page number indicates a figure or a table.

Ability language. *See also* Change talk
  evocative questions and, 142–143,
    142*t*
  overview, 8, 126, 127–128, 129
  questions to ask and, 11
  sustain talk and, 134*t*
Absolute worth, 20, 21, 24. *See also*
  Acceptance
Acceptance. *See also* PACE acronym
  affirmation and, 79
  client-centered approach and, 73
  genuineness and, 80
  influence and, 71
  overview, 19–24, 25
Accurate empathy. *See also* Empathy;
  Reflective listening
  ability language and, 127–128
  listening and, 32–33
  overview, 21–22, 24
Action stage of change, 10. *See also* Stages
  of change
Activation language, 132–133, 132*t*. *See
  also* Change talk
Active listening. *See* Listening; Reflective
  listening
Advice-giving stance. *See also* Advising
  evoking confidence and, 159–160
  listening and, 42
  overview, 13
  partnership and, 17–18
Advising, 91–94, 93*t*, 216. *See also* Advice-
  giving stance

Affirmation. *See also* Acceptance; OARS
  acronym (open-ended questions,
    affirmations, reflective listening, and
    summaries)
  agenda mapping and, 111
  confidence and, 160, 161*f*
  discord and, 190
  discrepancy and, 105
  engagement strategies and, 75
  evocation and, 147, 160, 161*f*
  overview, 24, 25, 79–82
  planning and, 111, 175–176
  supporting change and, 179
  understanding perspective and, 93–94,
    93*t*
Agency integration, 215–222
Agenda mapping, 109–113, 170–171. *See
  also* Focusing; Planning
Agreeing
  evocation and, 154–155
  listening and, 42
  planning and, 169
  reflective statements and, 87
  when to use motivational interviewing
    and, 48–55, 49*f*
Ambivalence
  evocation and, 28, 30, 134–138
  focusing and, 109
  overview, 100–103
  sustain talk and, 150, 182–183
  when to use motivational interviewing
    and, 49*f*, 50

Amplified reflection, 151–152. *See also* Reflections
Analyzing, 42
Anger
    interviewing methods and, 46
    responding to sustain talk and, 150
Apologizing, 190
Approach–approach form of ambivalence, 135. *See also* Ambivalence
Approach–avoidance form of ambivalence, 136. *See also* Ambivalence
Approval, 42
Argumentativeness, 45
Asking permission. *See* Permission asking
Assessment trap
    discord and, 187
    labeling trap and, 58–59
    overview, 56–57, 220
Attending, 35
Authority, 202–203
Autonomy. *See also* Acceptance; Choice
    addressing violations and sanctions and, 195
    evocation and, 153–154
    focusing and, 99–100
    neutrality and, 122
    overview, 22–23, 24, 241
    planning and, 174–175
Avoidance–avoidance form of ambivalence, 135. *See also* Ambivalence

B
Balance
    addressing violations and sanctions and, 193–196
    communication styles and, 68–71
    overview, 242
Barriers to change, 6–7. *See also* Change
Behavior and behavior change. *See also* Change
    addressing violations and sanctions, 191–197
    discrepancies and, 106–107
    fostering lasting change, 6–8
    as a goal, 2
    perceived obstacles and, 234
Benefits of change, 11
Blame
    blaming trap and, 59–61
    discord and, 184, 188
    listening and, 42
    overview, 204
Blended learning options, 226–230. *See also* Training

Booster sessions, 204
Brainstorming, 161

C
Change. *See also* Behavior and behavior change; Change talk; Stages of change
    ambivalence and, 100–103
    commitment and, 165–168
    drama of, 197–198
    evidence-based practice and, 4
    evocation and, 138
    fostering lasting change, 6–8
    as a goal, 2
    readiness for, 240
    supporting, 176, 178–179
    sustain talk and, 182–183
Change plan. *See* Planning
Change talk. *See also* Change
    ambivalence and discrepancy and, 134–138
    commitment and, 166
    evocation and, 138, 140–149, 142*t*
    overview, 8, 126–134, 132*t*, 134*t*, 183
    planning and, 165
    resistance and, 181–182
    responding to, 146–149
    supporting change and, 179
    training and, 216
Chat trap, 61
Check-in summaries, 10
Choice. *See also* Autonomy
    addressing violations and sanctions, 191–197
    autonomy-support and, 22
    neutrality and, 121–122, 123–124
    overview, 241
    perceived obstacles and, 234–236
Client Language EAsy Rating (CLEAR), 220
Client-centered style, 13, 71–74
Closed questions, 76–78
Coaching. *See also* Training
    blended learning options and, 226–230
    implementation of motivational interviewing programs and, 215
    overview, 218–219
    time involved in, 237–238
    training and, 216
Coding, 220–221
Coercion, 202–203
Cognitive-behavioral treatments, 213
Cognitive functioning, 89

Collaboration. *See also* Engagement;
  Partnership
  evocation and, 125, 139
  overview, 62–63
  perceived obstacles and, 233–234
  planning and, 165, 178–179
  questioning and, 78–79
  responding to sustain talk and, 150
  supporting change and, 178–179
Collecting summaries, 88–89. *See also*
  Summarizing
Coming alongside strategy, 156–157
Commitment. *See also* Change talk
  overview, 8, 130–131
  planning and, 165–168, 175–178,
    176–178
  questions to ask and, 11
  supporting change and, 179
  training and, 216
Communication
  advancing the interview, 51–55
  focusing and, 98
  open-ended questions and, 76–79
  problems with, 68–71
  stages of, 82–83, 83f
  styles of, 64–67, 65f, 66t
Communities of practice, 225–226,
  237–238
Compassion. *See also* PACE acronym
  affirmation and, 79
  client-centered approach and, 73
  discrepancy and, 105
  genuineness and, 80
  overview, 24–28
Complexity, 117
Compliance
  addressing violations and sanctions,
    191–197
  assessing, 241
  as a goal, 2
  overview, 16
  perceived obstacles and, 234–236
  punishment and incarceration and, 202
Condemnation, 71
Confidence
  evoking, 157, 158–163, 161f
  planning and, 175–176
  training and, 216
Confidence ruler, 159
Confidence talk strategy, 158–159
Conflict, 100–101
Confrontational approach
  addressing violations and sanctions and,
    194–195
  perceived obstacles and, 234

Consensus, 184
Contemplation stage of change, 10. *See
  also* Stages of change
Contingent relationships, 17
Continuum of change, 9–12, 9f. *See also*
  Change; Stages of change
Control
  compared to influence, 70–71
  listening and, 42
  partnership and, 17–18
  planning and, 171–172
Conversations. *See also* Interviewing
  methods
  advancing the interview, 51–55
  eliciting discussions, 109–115
  focusing and, 96–98, 109–115
  open-ended questions and, 76–79
  traps and, 55–61
Core correctional practice (CCP), 207
Correctional system, 19
Court system, 19
Crisis, 89
Criticism
  addressing violations and sanctions and,
    193–196
  labeling trap and, 58–59, 60
  listening and, 42
Curiosity, 147
Cynicism, 80

D

DARN acronym. *See also* Ability language;
    Desire language; Need language;
    Reason language
  evocative questions and, 142–143, 142t
  overview, 126
  sustain talk and, 133, 134t
DARN CATS acronym, 167
Decision making, 121–122
Defensiveness
  addressing violations and sanctions,
    191–192
  blaming trap and, 59–61
  discord and, 183–185, 188
  interviewing methods and, 45, 46
  overview, 13
Denial. *See also* Resistance
  addressing violations and sanctions and,
    196–197
  handling, 13–14
  perceived obstacles and, 233–234
Desire language. *See also* Change talk
  evocative questions and, 142–143,
    142t
  overview, 8, 126–127

questions to ask and, 11
    sustain talk and, 134*t*
Difficult situations, 192
Difficult topics, 118–119
Digital tools, 226–230
Directing communication style. *See also*
    Communication
    expert trap and, 69–70
    orienting and, 115
    overview, 64–67, 66*t*, 68–69
    planning and, 171–172
Directing conversations, 42
Disagreeing
    listening and, 42
    neutrality and, 120–124
    when to use motivational interviewing
        and, 48–55, 49*f*
Discomfort, 46
Discord. *See also* Resistance
    overview, 182, 183–186
    within the processes of motivational
        interviewing, 187–189
    responding to, 189–191
    role of the professional and, 186–
        187
    training and, 216
Discrepancy, 103–107, 134–138
Discussions, 109–115. *See also*
    Conversations
Disengagement, 186, 187–188. *See also*
    Engagement
Dishonesty
    addressing violations and sanctions,
        191–192
    discord and, 184
Distance learning, 226–230
Double approach–avoidance form
    of ambivalence, 136. *See also*
    Ambivalence
Double-sided reflection, 152, 153*t*. *See also*
    Reflections

E

Effective Practices in Community
    Supervision (EPICS), 213
Effectiveness of motivational interviewing,
    206, 219
Empathy. *See also* Accurate empathy;
    Reflective listening
    ability language and, 127–128
    affirmation and, 79
    client-centered approach and, 73
    genuineness and, 80
    listening and, 32–33
    overview, 21–22, 24

planning and, 174–175
    responding to sustain talk and,
        150
Engagement. *See also* Engagement
    strategies; Relationship with offenders
    affirmation and, 147
    client-centered approach and, 71–74
    commitment and, 166
    communication problems and, 68–71
    discord and, 186, 187–188
    overview, 62–64
    role of the professional and, 119–120
    styles of communication and, 64–67,
        65*f*, 66*t*
Engagement strategies. *See also*
    Engagement
    affirmation, 79–82
    asking open-ended questions, 76–79
    informing and advising, 91–94, 93*t*
    overview, 75
    preparing an offender for change and, 9
    reflection, 82–88, 83*f*, 84*t*
    summarizing, 88–91
Envisioning, 166
Ethics, 98–100, 122
Evidence-based practice, 4–6, 240
Evocation. *See also* Evocation strategies;
    PACE acronym
    ambivalence and discrepancy and,
        134–138
    change talk and, 126–134, 129, 132*t*,
        134*t*
    discord and, 188–189
    engagement and, 65*f*
    hope and confidence and, 157–163,
        161*f*
    with offender populations, 138–139
    overview, 28–30, 125
    planning and, 165
    training and, 216
Evocation strategies. *See also* Evocation
    eliciting change talk, 140–146, 142*t*
    overview, 140–141
    responding to change talk, 146–149
    responding to sustain talk, 149–157,
        153*t*
Evocative questions, 141–143, 142*t*. *See*
    also Evocation; Questions
Excuses, 13–14. *See also* Resistance
Experimentation, 166–167
Expert trap, 57, 69–70, 233–234
Extinction effect, 214–215
Extremes, considering, 143–145. *See also*
    Evocation
Eye contact, 35–36

F

Facial expressions, 36
Family relationships, 176–178
Feedback. *See also* Training
  implementation of motivational
    interviewing programs and,
    215
  overview, 218–219
  time involved in, 237–238
  training and, 216
Fidelity checks, 220–221
Focusing. *See also* Focusing strategies
  ambivalence and, 100–103
  discord and, 188, 190–191
  discrepancy and, 103–107
  engagement and, 65*f*
  overview, 95–98, 124
  values and ethics of, 98–100
Focusing strategies. *See also* Focusing
  clarifying goals, 115–120
  eliciting discussions, 109–115
  neutrality and, 120–124
  overview, 108, 124
Following communication style, 64–67,
    66*t*, 115. *See also* Communication
"Force over," 71. *See also* Control
Friendships, 176–178
Frustration, 105
Funding
  evidence-based practice and, 4–5
  implementation of motivational
    interviewing programs and, 214
Future hopes. *See* Hope

G

Genuineness
  affirmation and, 80–81, 81
  evocation and, 147
Goals
  clarifying, 115–120
  discrepancy and, 103–104, 106–
    107
  evocation and, 146
  focusing and, 96–98, 109–120, 115–
    120
  fostering lasting change and, 6–7
  neutrality and, 120–124
  planning and, 169–172, 173–174
  supporting change and, 179
  training and, 216
  when to use motivational interviewing
    and, 48–55, 49*f*
Guiding communication style, 64–67, 66*t*,
    115. *See also* Communication

H

Honesty. *See* Dishonesty
Hope
  evoking, 157–158
  training and, 216
Hopelessness, 27–28, 117
Hypothetical thinking strategy, 162–163

I

Implementation of motivational
    interviewing
  agency integration and, 215–222
  blended learning options and, 226–230
  communities of practice, 225–226
  informed practice and, 231–241
  overview, 211–215
  perceived obstacles, 231–241
  technologies and, 226–230
  train-the-trainer models, 222–225
Importance ruler, 143, 144. *See also*
    Evocation
Incarceration, 202–203
Influence, 70–71
Informed practice, 231–241
Informing
  evoking confidence and, 159–160
  overview, 91–94, 93*t*
  training and, 216
Integrated perspective, 101–102
Intention, 184
Interaction styles, 12–13
Interpreting
  listening and, 42
  reflective statements and, 85, 87
Interruption, 185
Interviewing methods
  advancing the interview, 51–55
  discord and, 187
  overview, 44–48, 61
  traps, 53, 55–61
  when to use motivational interviewing
    and, 48–55, 49*f*
Intrinsic motivations, 12–13, 23
Irritation, 46

J

Judgement
  absolute worth and, 21
  interviewing methods and, 46
  labeling trap and, 58–59, 60
  listening and, 32–33, 42
Justice, 100
Justice system, 19
Justification, 184

K

Key question, 90–91. *See also* Questions

L

Labeling trap, 58–59, 60, 188
Learning transfer, 215–222
Limitations, 175
Linking summaries, 89–90. *See also*
 Summarizing
Listening
 advancing the interview, 51–55
 communication and, 34–36, 66–67
 empathy and, 21–22
 instructions for, 32–34, 40–41, 41*f*
 necessity of, 31–32
 overview, 9, 31, 43
 reflective listening, 36–41, 37*t*, 38*t*, 40*t*,
  41*f*
 roadblocks to, 41–43
Logical stance, 13
Looking back/looking forward technique,
 145–146. *See also* Evocation

M

Maintenance stage of change, 10. *See also*
 Stages of change
Masquerade question, 77. *See also* Closed
 questions; Questions
Meditation, 32–33
Methods, interviewing. *See* Interviewing
 methods
MI Skills Code (MISC), 220
MI Treatment Integrity (MITI), 220–221
Mindfulness, 32–33
Minimizing, 184
Mobilizing change talk. *See also* Change
 talk
 discrepancy and, 137–138
 sustain talk and, 133–134, 134*t*
 taking steps language, 133–134, 134*t*
Moralizing, 42
Motivation in general, 72
Motivational interviewing in general. *See*
 also Interviewing methods
 concerns regarding, 207–210, 209*t*
 core correctional practice (CCP) and,
  207–210, 209*t*
 with offender populations, 201–210,
  209*t*
 overview, 3–14, 9*f*, 15–16, 44, 47–48,
  199–201, 207–210, 209*t*, 241–
  242
Motivational speech, 8. *See also* Change
 talk

N

Need for change, 143. *See also* Preparatory
 change talk
Need language. *See also* Change talk
 evocative questions and, 142–143, 142*t*
 overview, 8, 126, 129–130
 sustain talk and, 134*t*
Neutrality, 120–124, 194–195. *See also*
 Focusing
Noncompliance, 191–197. *See also*
 Compliance
Nonverbal cues, 35–36, 40–41, 41*f*,
 206
"Not-knowing" stance, 57

O

OARS acronym (open-ended questions,
 affirmations, reflective listening, and
 summaries). *See also* Affirmation;
 Open-ended questions; Reflective
 listening; Summarizing
 agenda mapping and, 111
 evocation and, 147–149
 orienting and, 115
 overview, 75
 training and, 216
Obstacles to MI, 231–241
Open-ended questions. *See also* OARS
 acronym (open-ended questions,
 affirmations, reflective listening, and
 summaries); Questions
 agenda mapping and, 111
 engagement strategies and, 75
 evocation and, 147
 overview, 76–79
Opposition
 discord and, 185
 responding to sustain talk and, 150
Orienting, 113–115. *See also* Focusing
Outcomes, 206, 219

P

PACE acronym. *See also* Acceptance;
 Compassion; Evocation;
 Partnership
 affirmation and, 79
 overview, 16
 perceived obstacles and, 233–234
 training and, 216
Partnership. *See also* Engagement; PACE
 acronym
 affirmation and, 79
 genuineness and, 80
 overview, 16–19

Passivity
    discord and, 187
    interviewing methods and, 46
    perceived obstacles and, 236–237
Peer learning, 225–226. *See also* Training
Permission asking
    advising and, 91–92
    focusing and, 119
    planning and, 171
Person-centered approach, 47
Perspective, 92–94, 93*t*
Planning
    from change talk to, 165
    commitment and, 165–168, 176–178
    discord and, 188, 189
    engagement and, 65*f*
    overview, 164
    preparing an offender for change and,
        9
    process of, 168–172, 173–174
    roadblocks to, 172, 174–176
    supporting change and, 176, 178–179
    training and, 216
Power, 83–84, 202–203
"Power with," 71. *See also* Influence
Powerlessness
    interviewing methods and, 46
    praise and, 81
Practice, 34, 216
Praise
    compared to affirmation, 81
    listening and, 42
Precision tuning, 115. *See also* Orienting
Precontemplation stage of change, 10. *See
    also* Stages of change
Premature focus trap, 58–59, 118–119. *See
    also* Focusing
Preparation of organizational change,
        213–214. *See also* Implementation of
        motivational interviewing
Preparation stage of change, 10. *See also*
    Stages of change
Preparatory change talk. *See also* Ability
        language; Change talk; Desire
        language; Need language; Reason
        language
    ability language and, 127–128
    activation language and, 132–133, 132*t*
    discrepancy and, 137–138
    evocation and, 143, 147
    need language and, 130
    overview, 126
Preparing for change, 8–12, 9*f. See also*
    Change

Problem solving
    compared to planning, 168–169
    preparing an offender for change and, 9
Productive talk, 9
Professional listening, 40–41, 41*f. See also*
    Listening
Professional relationship. *See* Relationship
    with offenders
Program implementation. *See*
    Implementation of motivational
    interviewing
Progress monitoring, 241
Punishment, 202–203

Q

Querying extremes, 143–145. *See also*
    Evocation
Questions. *See also* Open-ended questions
    commitment and, 166
    communication styles and, 66–67
    evocation and, 141–143, 142*t*
    interviewing methods and, 46–47
    listening and, 42
    overview, 10–12
    reflective statements and, 83–84, 84*f*, 87
    summarizing and, 90–91

R

Rationalizations, 13–14. *See also*
    Resistance
Readiness to change, 240. *See also* Change;
    Stages of change
Reason language. *See also* Change talk
    evocation and, 142–143, 142*t*, 146–147
    overview, 8, 126, 128–129
    sustain talk and, 134*t*
Reflections. *See also* Reflective listening
    agenda mapping and, 111
    evocation and, 148, 151–152, 153*t*
    overview, 10, 82–88, 83*f*, 84*t*
    planning and, 174–175
    reflective listening and, 38*t*, 39–41, 40*t*,
        41*f*
    responding to sustain talk and,
        149–157, 153*t*
    supporting change and, 178–179
Reflective listening. *See also* Accurate
        empathy; Listening; OARS acronym
        (open-ended questions, affirmations,
        reflective listening, and summaries);
        Reflections
    engagement and, 75, 82–88, 83*f*, 84*t*
    evocation and, 148
    instructions for, 40–41, 41*f*

overview, 36–41, 37t, 38t, 40t, 41f, 82–83, 83f
responding to sustain talk and, 149–157, 153t
strategic responses, 153–157
training and, 216
Reframing, 154–155, 161–162. *See also* Evocation
Rehabilitation, 204
Relationship with offenders. *See also* Engagement; Therapeutic alliance
affirmation and, 147
client-centered approach and, 71–74
core correctional practice (CCP) and, 207
discord and, 189–191
overview, 205–206
supporting change and, 178–179
Relationships with others, 176–178
Repetition, 38–39, 38t
Resentment, 150
Resistance. *See also* Discord
addressing violations and sanctions, 191–197
commitment and, 166
evocation and, 28
handling, 13–14
overview, 150, 180–182
sustain talk and, 181–183
Resolve, 166
Resources available to offenders, 175
Respect, 80, 81
Responsibility
addressing violations and sanctions and, 195
blaming trap and, 59–61
for change, 12–13
partnership and, 19
Restrictions, 175
Reviewing past successes strategy, 160
Rhetorical question, 77. *See also* Closed questions; Questions
Righting reflex
discord and, 188
expert trap and, 69
overview, 55–56, 181
perceived obstacles and, 234
premature focus trap and, 58
Risk–needs–responsivity (RNR) model, 5–6, 202–203, 213
Role of the professional
addressing violations and sanctions, 192–193
discord and, 186–187

evocation and, 139
explaining to offenders, 192–193
focusing and, 119–120
overview, 203–206
planning and, 169
Running head start strategy, 155–156

S

Sanctions
addressing, 191–197
instituting, 241
Science-based methods, 5
Self-deception, 184
Self-directed change, 2. *See also* Change
Self-exploration
discrepancy and, 105–107
evocation and, 138
listening and, 41–42
Shame
discrepancy and, 105
influence and, 71
interviewing methods and, 46
Shifting focus, 190–191. *See also* Focusing
Silent absorbing, 40–41, 41f
Smoke alarms. *See* Discord
Solutions, 42
Staff Training Aimed at Reducing Re-arrest (STARR), 213
Stages of change. *See also* Change
overview, 9–12, 9f
readiness to change and, 240
when to use motivational interviewing and, 50
Status quo, 182
Straight reflection, 151. *See also* Reflections
Strategic Training Initiative in Community Supervision (STICS), 213
Strengths. *See also* Strengths-based approaches
evoking confidence and, 160, 161f
focusing and, 109–115
planning and, 171–172
Strengths-based approaches. *See also* Strengths
affirmation and, 81
evocation and, 28, 29–30
Stuckness
ambivalence and, 102
focusing and, 117–118
Suggestions, 42

Summarizing. *See also* OARS acronym
    (open-ended questions, affirmations,
    reflective listening, and summaries)
  agenda mapping and, 111
  engagement strategies and, 75
  evocation and, 148–149
  overview, 88–91
  supporting change and, 179
Supervision, 217–218, 225–226. *See also*
    Training
Supportive stance, 13, 105
Sustain talk
  ambivalence and discrepancy and,
    134–138
  commitment and, 167
  evocation and, 138
  overview, 126–134, 132*t*, 134*t*
  resistance and, 181–183
  responding to, 149–157, 153*t*
  supporting change and, 179
  training and, 216
Sustainability, 211, 221–222, 230

T

Tag question, 77. *See also* Closed
    questions; Questions
Taking steps language, 133–134, 134*t*. *See
    also* Change talk
Talking, 33–34
Teaching
  listening and, 42
  partnership and, 17–18
Technology, 226–230
Teleconferencing, 228
Telling
  listening and, 42
  partnership and, 17–18
  planning and, 171–172
Therapeutic alliance. *See also* Engagement;
    Relationship with offenders
  overview, 62–63
  questioning and, 78–79
  role of the professional and, 119–
    120
Thinking for a Change (T4C), 213
Threatening, 193–196
Time involved, 237–238

Training
  agency integration and, 215–222
  blended learning options, 226–230
  communities of practice and, 225–226
  implementation of motivational
    interviewing programs and, 214, 215
  overview, 212–213
  time involved in, 237–238
  train-the-trainer models, 222–225
Transitional summaries, 90–91. *See also*
    Summarizing
Truthfulness. *See* Dishonesty

U

Understanding
  ability language and, 127–128
  the offender's perspective, 92–94, 93*t*
  reflective statements and, 83–84
Undivided attention, 35. *See also* Attending

V

Validation, 24. *See also* Acceptance;
    Affirmation
Values
  discrepancy and, 103–104, 106–107
  evocation and, 146
  focusing and, 98–100, 109–115
  responsibility for change and, 12–13
Video Assessment of Simulated
    Encounters-Revised (VASE-R),
    220–221
Videoconferencing, 228
Violations, 191–197
Visual aids, 113

W

Web conferencing, 228–229
Web courses and webinars, 229–230
"Why" question, 78. *See also* Closed
    questions; Questions
Withdrawing, 42
Working relationship, 62–63. *See also*
    Engagement; Relationship with
    offenders
Workshop training, 216–217. *See also*
    Training
Worth, absolute. *See* Absolute worth